IGNORANCE

AND FEAR

A Personal Battle Against Bowel Cancer

Why Not Me?

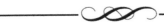

Anthony Michaels

This book is dedicated to a number of people.

I would like to thank my loved ones for helping and

supporting me on my journey.

Words are never enough to express how much that meant.

CONTENTS

those who have looked after me on my journey and begin life once more, after over a year of being a victim of cancer. I am much less ignorant of the UK's second biggest cancer killer than I was before my 'journey' began.

I would like to thank all the professionals who brought my journey to an end as I had always hoped. Mr Syed, Doctor Patel, Katherine, Louise and Fiona: you all acted so professionally and were so caring whilst I was under your care. I thank you now and will do so for a lifetime. (Naturally, these professionals' names have been changed to protect their identity.)

My greatest thank you goes to my wife who was by my side through each step of this journey.

Two people 'I know' inspired me to write this book: Sarah and Sophie. Sarah is, undoubtedly one of the bravest people I have ever had the pleasure of meeting. She has been through numerous journeys despite her young age. Sarah, you truly are a 'Wonder Woman.'

Sophie, I have never met you but, despite that, you inspired me to continue writing and to complete this book. You are on your journey even though you are so young. My thoughts will be with you throughout.

May your hearts beat strong, always.

PREFACE

The author, Anthony Michaels, writes a personal account of his experience, prior to and after diagnosis of the UK's second biggest cancer killer: bowel cancer. For some, this is still a taboo subject. The reader is taken on his 'journey' from initial symptoms to subsequent medical investigations, surgery, infection and, ultimately, a challenging chemotherapy regime. His words are engaging and written by a 'real' person and not by a medical expert, making them easy to relate to. The experiences he endured are described intimately, with feeling and, surprisingly, with humour when appropriate.

He tells in intimate detail exactly what persuaded him to seek medical help, the fear relating to those initial medical visits and how medical staff helped and supported him on each step of his harrowing journey. The reader learns how these experiences affected not only him, but those dearest to him, and how the kindness of close friends eased his anguish.

Mr. Michaels allows the reader an insight into this cruellest of illnesses, how cancer weaved its vicious web and the treatment used to fight against it.

He describes how, prior to diagnosis, he had very little knowledge of any cancer, let alone bowel cancer, and the words he has written allow the reader to be less ignorant and fearful of the symptoms and treatment accompanying this disease. After all, we know that often ignorance breeds fear, and the author's words help to alleviate some of those fears.

Much of the book deals with the six months of chemotherapy treatment which he endured but he was not just shut in a room and left to suffer the consequences of the liquid flowing through his veins. The doctors and other medical staff listened to his concerns and could see the effects the treatment was having upon his body, resulting in the medical experts helping to nurse him through the side-effects he suffered: from the feelings of sickness to the sleepless nights and loss of hair from some surprising parts of his body. Aside from the many other side-effects, it details advice from those looking after him about what he should and shouldn't eat, what pastimes he should and shouldn't undertake, and how his body may or may not react. These reactions are unknown until the treatment has commenced, so some very unusual occurrences are possible, and the author certainly experiences his fair share of them!

Bowel cancer, undoubtedly, changed the author's life and this is reflected in his words. The experience is described candidly. No punches are pulled with questions being posed and answered.

We all know that cancer does not discriminate. It affects young and old, black and white, gay or straight, absolutely anyone. A question many will ask is: 'Why me?' when the question one should actually ask is 'Why not me?' When the reader poses this question, then Mr. Michaels' words may well offer some comfort should they be given a cancer diagnosis.

INTRODUCTION

I began writing this book because the words 'bowel cancer,' literally, meant very little to me. Until I was diagnosed with this awful disease, I was extremely ignorant of it. To me it was something that would happen to others and by-pass me. Why is that? The problem with us, as human beings, can be the way we think. For example, this will happen to someone else and it won't happen to me. It is acceptable to think like that about many things and that way of thinking may well be correct about many of those things. With cancer it is not. You should not think that you will not be diagnosed with cancer during your lifetime because there is as much chance that you will as there is that you won't. Instead of thinking to yourself 'it won't happen to me' think to yourself, 'why won't it happen to me?' If you can answer that question, you should immediately contact all the pharmaceutical companies on the planet, along with all the medical professionals dealing with cancer, and let them know that they can stop their work. You can then inform them of why you will never be diagnosed with cancer and, I guarantee, you will become a billionaire, almost overnight.

Prior to my diagnosis, I did not know what procedures I would have to endure, what treatment may follow or how long that treatment would be necessary. No one told me that a surgeon may not even pick up a scalpel whilst he was operating on me but sit at a screen whilst a large robot standing nearby, its numerous metal arms outstretched, cut into me. No one told me about the many different kinds of chemotherapy treatment there were and how this kind of treatment could affect my body and my mind. I knew nothing of this treatment, what it involved, how long it went on for or what happens when it's completed.

Prior to diagnosis, I knew that if you had blood in your poo you should get it checked and that was it. That was, literally, all I knew about this kind of cancer. I never saw any advertisements on the television, or heard any on the radio, regarding bowel cancer. I did not know of anyone who had died from bowel cancer, recovered from it or currently suffered from it. That can't be right, can it? I mean this kind of cancer is so common and becoming more prevalent, with vast numbers of people being diagnosed with it each year. Oh, and by the way, those numbers are rapidly rising.

Obviously, I heard that 'so and so' had died of cancer or 'he or she' had been diagnosed with cancer, but no one, ever, said 'bowel cancer', they just said 'cancer.' I heard of people dying of skin cancer, breast cancer or lung cancer but, never, ever bowel cancer. If it wasn't mentioned, then people, naturally, wouldn't talk of it, wouldn't ask questions and, when it happened to them, would know very little about what they were facing.

I have a very small circle of friends and people I know. Out of this circle I know of three individuals that were diagnosed with bowel cancer. That's three out of a very small number. One individual suffered from it twice! Another died from it and the other made a recovery. Out of those three, I only knew that two had been diagnosed with it long after they were treated. They were not old people, I can assure you. The lady who sadly passed away was only fifty-one!

Bowel cancer is extremely common and is, in fact, the UK's second biggest cancer killer, yet I knew almost nothing about it. Now I do. Let me give you an example. A work colleague approached me one day, clearly worried about something. He had heard that I had suffered from bowel cancer and because of that, felt he could approach me. He explained that he had noticed a small amount of blood coming from his anus. Clearly it was a huge worry to him, so much so that he aired his fears to me, someone he barely knew. I immediately asked him what colour the blood was. Was it very dark in colour, almost brown, or lighter? He replied that it was not dark, more of a lighter colour. Although I had and have no medical expertise and absolutely no medical training whatsoever, that was enough information for me to guess, almost instantly, that he didn't have a major problem, and I encouraged him to visit his doctor. He did and it turned out he had piles. Next time he has that problem, he will not be as ignorant and fearful. We all know that ignorance breeds fear.

My words are written as a normal, everyday person, those of a patient and in layman's terms. They are the words as they were told to me during my treatment and I do not speak in medical terms, but as a member of the public who has been diagnosed with this cruel illness. I have written my words truthfully and have not pulled any punches. I see no point in viewing my experiences through 'rose tinted glasses'. Simply put, it was what it was.

Hopefully by the time you have read this book you will have learnt a few things and be less ignorant and certainly less fearful.

A.M.

CHAPTER ONE

Problems

The year 2015 began as any 'normal' year. Winter passed, spring sprang and summer, well, that was like any other British summer; the weather was less than perfect, shall we say. We carried on as though it was the greatest summer, weather-wise, there had ever been, just like we did through all the British summers I could remember. My forty-eighth birthday came and went.

I was working for a small, independently owned business as I had done so for a number of years and had reached the dizzy heights of management. It was a stressful occupation and my working hours could be long. Although I had not enjoyed the work I was undertaking for some time, the pay was good and afforded me, my wife, our seventeen-year-old son and our favourite kind of canine friend, a Bassett Hound named Benson, a decent standard of living. My daughter and granddaughter lived close by, some fifteen-minute drive away, and were frequent visitors to our house.

Two major events occurred during September that year. Firstly, it was our beautiful granddaughter's first birthday and, secondly, my mother-in-law, the lovely Jean, was diagnosed with terminal cancer. Jean was your typical wife, mother, grandmother and great-grandmother. She doted on her children, grandchildren and great-granddaughter. She was always full of life, usually with a smile on her face.

Whilst our children were young, she was always on-hand, offering a helping hand and, more times than not, able to look after them at extremely short notice, without question. She loved children. Being surrounded by them was a pleasure, so much so that she became a registered childminder. Often, whilst visiting, there would be numerous children of varying ages playing and squabbling together in her front room which had been converted into a nursery. She looked after the children whilst my wife's father would be pottering around the rear garden or fiddling with whatever current automobile was in the driveway. Their house was always a welcoming home and I never had any reservations about visiting.

Jean loved a party! An annual knees-up always took place at her house. Jean and my father-in-law would invite as many of the neighbours as possible and most obliged. On these occasions, my wife and I would arrive and the door was opened by people we had never even seen, let alone met! It was not abnormal for such events to continue until the small hours. Food and drink would always be plentiful. Beers and spirits were consumed along with supplies of homemade chilli con carnie and curries.

Approximately a month prior to her terminal diagnosis, Jean became very ill. She was unable to eat and felt generally unwell. Numerous doctor and hospital visits followed, resulting in her diagnosis, cancer, which had spread into her bones. The doctors decided that a course of radiotherapy may help. It didn't. Treatment was ceased and we all waited for the inevitable. Pain management was the only option left. Naturally, this was a devastating blow to her family, friends and those close to her.

Christmas 2015 approached rapidly and Jean was clearly struggling. Her cancer had clearly spread further and she would sit on her couch in her living room, vacantly staring ahead, before fiddling with some imaginary item she thought she was holding in her hands. Only she was able to see what was in her grasp. She wore a pump discretely about her person, which would activate almost hourly, releasing morphine into her bloodstream in an attempt to ease her suffering. Community nurses visited several times a day, helping her as best they could, but everyone, apart from Jean, knew what the result would be.

Jean was now extremely weak, losing a huge amount of weight and becoming unstable on her feet, falling over on numerous occasions. Her falls often resulted in broken bones leading to numerous weeks spent in the hospital.

When visiting her, Jean would often hurl abuse at her loved ones, something I had never seen her do before her illness. It was shocking and unnerving to experience, seeing such a change in someone so full of life and love. It was as though a demon had taken over her mind which was true in so many ways.

Abuse was hurled at her husband. She would accuse him

of all manner of things, none of which were true. She thought people were trying to kill her and steal her possessions which was again so far from the truth. It was very sad to see all this happening to her, so heart-breaking for her loved ones to experience, but what could be done? The demon had now taken over her mind and the cancer had spread into the farthest corners of her body and, quite clearly, into her brain. As 'He' travelled through her, 'He' destroyed each part 'He' touched, leaving parts of her broken, unrepairable, until 'He' needed to travel no more. It now became a waiting game.

It was around December 2015 that I too began experiencing changes to my own body. I had never been seriously ill and had only ever spent one night in hospital, having undergone an operation on my nose, the result of cricket ball meeting my nose which caused breakage and blockage. My first wife decided that, due to the resulting high decibel snoring which followed this unfortunate collision, we should sleep in separate rooms which would continue until the blockage was removed, hence my operation. By the time the procedure had taken place, we had gone our separate ways and I had just met the current Mrs Michaels, who reminds me almost daily, that the 'operation didn't work!'

Following the breaking of my nose, I suffered several broken bones due to my ineptitude at playing a certain sport but I had never been seriously ill.

I was always a creature of habit, just as most of the human race are. I would wake in the morning, shower, dress and make that first cup of coffee which would kick start my day. Having rushed my first cup of coffee, purely so I could I had time for another, I would visit the toilet and open my bowels. It was as though the caffeine had rushed its way through my body into my vital organs, setting off a rapid chain of events, culminating in me sitting on my 'throne'. It had been that way for as long as I could remember. It was normal for me and may well be for you. What wasn't normal was what I began to excrete.

I began sitting on my 'throne' more often. Whereas one visit had always been sufficient to see me through to the next morning, it was now not the case. It was as though, during the first sitting, I was only able to empty part of what was lurking in my bowels. One sitting just wasn't enough! I began to notice some discolouration in what was leaving me and, over the course of days, it became darker. It continued altering in colour, becoming almost black. I did what a lot of males of our species would do. I continued, hoping it would go away. Guess what? It didn't.

Christmas came and went and during January 2016 further changes took place. Blood had clearly appeared within my stools. As much as I wanted to believe differently, it was unmistakeable. Even a blind person would have seen it.

I was visiting the toilet more and more, less faeces being discharged with each sitting. I continued on my merry way hoping, beyond hope, that everything would return to normal, burying my head in the sand. As the weeks passed, rapid changes began to take place. I was now visiting the toilet around ten times a day. February came and went. With the passing of February, I began suffering stomach cramps.

They came without warning and, although infrequent, took my breath away. Cramps were followed by the inevitable 'throne' visits, but what I was passing had changed. It had become what resembled a mixture of blood, mucus and faeces. The blood was very dark in colour and I was passing something which I would describe as resembling the white of a freshly cracked egg. It was similar in texture, but a very dark, reddish, brown colour.

By now, controlling my bowels had become more difficult. One morning, whilst sitting in front of my desk at work, I suffered a severe stomach cramp which resulted in me dashing to the lavatory. I entered the small room, barely having time to flick the light switch, before undoing and dropping my trousers and underwear. My heart was pounding as happens in these situations.

As I stood, my knees slightly bent, about to assume the sitting position, some of the discoloured 'egg white' escaped my body, landing on the previously clean, tiled floor next to the white enamel of the toilet. Luckily nothing else followed! Momentarily, I examined what had landed on the floor, wishing I was elsewhere. It was very bloodied and around two inches in length and was the texture of raw egg white. I felt that had I closed my thumb and forefinger over one end of it and pulled, the rest would have slithered along the floor, following what I had grasped between my two digits and remaining joined together. I was shocked by what had occurred, as anyone else would have been. Luckily, I was alone! I cleaned up the mess I had made, cleaned my posterior and returned to my work position. Outwardly, I probably appeared normal. Inside, I was feeling anything but.

March arrived and Jean had gone from home to hospital and was now resident in a care home. She was bedridden, her bed placed against the window so she could view the ocean. The view was lovely, with ships and smaller vessels going about their journeys, although at times it was doubtful Jean understood what she was seeing. My wife and I visited regularly. She was now at a stage where she was losing weight almost daily and had become extremely weak. It was as though anyone could have walked into her room and scooped her up in their arms, lifting her from the mattress.

Jean was now being more abusive than ever. My father-in-law would arrive and immediately the words would flow from her pale lips.

'You've been with that woman, haven't you John?' she would blurt out. My father-in-law would look at me quizzically and I would return his look with equal disbelief.

'I've seen you both together, holding hands! You've been outside with her and I caught you.' Her remarks would be full of scorn and mainly aimed towards her husband, the man who had been by her side, slept next to her, lived with her through so many years. I felt nothing but sorrow for this poor woman. In her mind, she believed in what she was saying and was totally convinced by what she had seen. In what had become her world, it was completely real and no matter how you tried to convince her otherwise, it was a fruitless task. Then, as if by magic, the abuse would cease as quickly as it began and a small piece of the old Jean would briefly emerge before she drifted off to sleep, unable to fight the weakness which consumed her.

This abuse was, now, all too common and we became used to it. We knew that what was spewing from Jean's mouth was total fabrication and the only person who believed it was the person saying it. This made the outbursts all the sadder. There were no actions or words we could find to explain why this demon made Jean think or say these things.

The whole family had become emotionally drained by what had occurred during the space of the last six months or so. We had seen this lovely woman turn from a fun, life-loving, caring and physically fit person to someone who was now broken both mentally and in body. She had descended more and more rapidly to the point of no return. Abuse would be hurled at her loved ones and then, as if a switch had been flicked, she would tell you how much she loved and cared for you.

Whenever her great-granddaughter visited, her face would light up and she would hold out a thin hand lovingly, just wanting to hold the child tightly, but she was unable, physically to do so.

By now I never really saw Jean in any noticeable pain. This was being managed by the drugs being pumped into her system. She would wake, smile, hurl the abuse, visualise something that was non-existent and then rest.

Much of the time, Jean would imagine that she was lying in a cabin on a large, magnificent cruise liner with a view of some far-flung land. Prior to her illness, she had loved travelling on cruise ships to warmer climes with loved ones and when she took in the view from her window she could, somehow, see through the driving rain and howling wind into another world, a world, where she was in her 'heaven'.

My wife was being very brave under the circumstances, but I could also see her suffering. Naturally, she was devastated by what had happened to her beloved mother. I had told her about my 'ailment' but not the full extent. I felt she was undergoing enough suffering with her own mother's rapid decline and I kept the finer details of my situation near to my heart.

Naturally, my problems continued and it was apparent they weren't going to cease of their own accord. Around this time, I recall an incident whilst I was at work. By now, I was visiting the toilet in excess of ten times per day, mainly passing a mixture of dark red blood, 'egg white' and faeces. I found myself cleaning the area frequently and, sometimes, the liquid would seep from me without warning. It was not enough for me to soil myself, but, from the feeling around the area, I knew it was present and needed wiping away.

One afternoon, whilst at work, and having cleaned myself on numerous occasions throughout the day, I happened to walk past one of the secretaries who was sitting at her desk. I had known this particular secretary for more than twenty years and she was not known for her tactfulness. Within a second of me passing her desk, she stopped typing, looked up from her desk and exclaimed:

'You stink!'

This remark alerted another secretary sitting close by who retorted:

'What of?'

I didn't hear any further conversation between the secretaries as I scurried embarrassingly from the room, straight to the lavatory. Upon lowering my trousers and underwear to my knees, I was relieved to discover that my underwear was not soiled. Again, I cleaned myself and the all too common mixture of dark blood, faeces and 'egg white' was present.

I returned to my desk. My pride was almost reduced to zero and my embarrassment levels had risen uncontrollably to new heights. That same afternoon I did what I should have done around four months earlier and made that dreaded telephone call to the local health centre and an appointment was made to see my General Practitioner.

I had known this day would come, but I had delayed as long as I could. Now there was no turning back. The reason for the delay was a simple one. Ignorance and fear. I didn't know what my problem was exactly and feared what would be discovered. Knowing what I know now, I would have turned the clock back several months without hesitation.

Several days later, I was sitting in the waiting room of the town's health centre. It was now late March and my forty-ninth birthday had passed. Upon my arrival, I checked in and visited the toilet to make sure I was 'presentable' to the doctor; after all, first impressions last! As I sat on one of the approximately thirty chairs lined up in the waiting room, waiting for the electronic information board to instruct me to go to Dr Richardson's room, I began to reflect.

It was now late March and I had been suffering my problems for around three to four months. I recalled how my wife, for some time, had urged me to visit the doctor. My work colleagues now knew I was suffering from some sort of stomach ailment but I had kept the majority of the gory details from all of them. Naturally, I had confided in my wife more than I had my work colleagues but not to any great extent. Had my ailment been to my toe or finger, I would have been much more willing to be completely open with them!

I had an extremely good friend at work whom I had told more about my suffering than any of my other work colleagues. Patrick and I had known each other most of our working lives and had both joined our present employer in our early twenties. Patrick was a couple of years younger than me and a few inches shorter than my six-foot frame! He had very dark brown hair and was strikingly handsome. He reminded me of a young Keanu Reeves with his good looks and his slightly tanned complexion. He was also blessed with 'the gift of the gab,' knowing what to say and when to say it. It was easy to be envious of his good looks and social skills and, to some extent, I was.

We became extremely good friends over the years and when a problem arose, we were able to confide in each other. He knew I was ill but, due to the nature of my problems, I felt unable to tell even him their extent.

I thought about my children. My daughter was now approaching her twenty-first birthday and my son his seventeenth. I was looking forward to their special days and I found it helpful to have something good to focus on in the future: something that was pleasant, which momentarily stopped me thinking of my current journey.

Most of my thoughts were of my lovely wife. I was a year older than her and we had married whilst in our late twenties. Everything had run smoothly for around ten years, but I had thought, for some reason, that I was missing out on some aspects of life. This led to us parting for approximately six years. I won't go into the details as they are irrelevant to this book, but we found ourselves back together in 2011, some years prior to the beginning of my problems. We are together now and I want nothing more than for that to remain the case. It may be a cliché, but the grass certainly is not always greener on the other side!

My wife was now under extreme emotion, although she hid it as best she could. Her mother was gravely ill, having only weeks or days left in this world, and her husband was now ill. I was glad I was able to keep some of my gory details from her.

My train of thought was interrupted by my name appearing in flashing lights on the electronic notice board hanging on the wall of the surgery.

'Anthony Michaels, please go to Dr Richardson's room' it read. I rose and, in my thoughts, walked confidently to another uncomfortable seat outside the doctor's room. Within seconds the door swung inwards and Dr Richardson stood in the doorway. She was in her early forties with light brown, curly, shoulder-length hair. She had a slight smile on her face and introduced herself. Before I had time to speak, she raised her right forefinger, as if pointing to the ceiling, and exclaimed a little excitedly, 'You've come for this!'

'Have I?' I replied with the first words I could think of.

She could obviously see that I was nervous and, having invited me into her office, attempted to put me at ease with small talk. Having explained my symptoms to her, some of which had she had clearly been told when I made the appointment, she invited me to drop my trousers and underwear. I then bent over, my hands against the mattress of the bed, which was pushed against the wall. She explained what I was about to undergo would be 'slightly uncomfortable' and I heard the sound of plastic against skin, as she put at least one rubber glove on.

Within seconds she had completed her work. She was correct, the procedure was only 'slightly uncomfortable'. Had it been a male doctor, it may have been more uncomfortable due to the extra length and girth of the male finger! Although the procedure was disconcerting, it really was no big deal. 'Slightly uncomfortable' was exactly the correct way of describing it. Dr

Richardson explained that whilst she had been 'intimate' with me she had found nothing untoward and she would arrange for me to have a 'flexible sigmoidoscopy'. Basically, in layman's terms, that's a camera up your arse!

I was given some paperwork by the doctor and she urged me to call the telephone number displayed on the documentation so the appointment could be made. She then said her farewells, commenting that I shouldn't worry about our intimacy as I probably would not see her again. I replied that we may bump into each other in the local supermarket. She smiled and I left. We never did bump into each other. My journey had now begun.

I did as advised and telephoned to make an appointment for my 'camera action' and one was received. I can't recall exactly when my appointment was set but it was around ten days after my meeting with Dr Richardson. It was to be undertaken in a neighbouring town some five miles from where I lived.

I continued working, even though I had now become tired and lethargic. My ten-a-day-plus visits to the toilet continued and my stomach cramps began to increase in frequency. All these things prompted me in a new course of action.

When I was promoted to manager, I was given certain perks, as can be customary. My boss had increased my wages but had also included me in the company's private medical insurance scheme. Until now I had no need for it. I recalled how my boss had proudly told me that the company would pay the premiums, adding that it wasn't only necessarily for my benefit but also for the benefit of the company as it would allow me to recover more quickly from any illness so I could return to work promptly.

As I had never needed the use of private medical insurance before, I was slightly apprehensive of the procedure. I needn't have worried. Now I had visited my GP and nothing had been found, the shackles, so to speak, were off. I had experienced my first real 'intimate' procedure and, like many things, the thought of undertaking it had been far worse than the actual undertaking. Don't get me wrong, to me it wasn't a pleasant experience, but it wasn't as bad as I'd assumed it would be. Dr Richardson was very professional and had put me at ease with her reassurance. It didn't bother me at all that the doctor was female. Female, male or hermaphrodite – it did not matter as long as they could help me.

So, with my internal examination providing no results, I made the arrangements to be treated privately. The insurers supplied me with an account number and the details of the nearest hospital I was permitted to visit. A short telephone call later and I was booked in for a consultation. This was to take place during the afternoon on Monday 4th April 2016 with Professor Shamari. My initial telephone call to the insurers took place on 31st March 2016.

I was now feeling much happier, happier than at any time during the last four months. The ball was now rolling and, finally, after so much uncertainty, I began to gain confidence. Officially I didn't know what my condition was, although I knew cancer was a possibility, along with a number of other illnesses. At least now, as each day passed, I was getting nearer to the truth. Once the truth was known, something could be done about it.

CHAPTER TWO

The End of the Suffering

During the early hours of 2nd April 2016, my wife received a telephone call from her father. Even before he relayed the news, my wife and I both instinctively knew what it was. The demon that was Mr C had eventually finished 'His' work on Jean's body and mind. It had been approximately seven months in the making. 'He' had gone about 'His' work rapidly and deliberately, reducing 'His' subject from someone healthy in both body and mind to someone bedridden, weighing around five stone. Mr C had taken her body, then her mind, stealing her without mercy from those who loved her.

Even though we knew this day would, inevitably, arrive, the pain was no less. We left our home to visit Jean. My father-in-law was there by her side, as he had been when she slipped away. He had been called to the home and arrived, literally, minutes before she was taken. He had spoken to her, saying those words that only someone who had been married for fifty years could say. As he did so, he explained that a tear had left Jean's closed right eye, running down her cheek and onto her pillow. In that instant, she was gone. She left behind a husband, two daughters, a son, six grandchildren and one great-granddaughter, along with someone who would probably miss her the most, her mother.

I had now seen, first hand, how cancer operated. It was as though 'He' made 'Himself' invisible, disguised 'Himself' inside Jean, until 'He' decided to make an appearance. It seemed to be 'His' choice when that moment should be. 'His' task with Jean had now been completed. The disgusting work 'He' began, just a short time earlier, was now finished and it was time to move on, to infect some other poor soul and continue the task, destroying another life and affecting, beyond words, all those connected to that life. 'His' work was disgusting and the way it was carried out was evil and without mercy. Cancer chose without thought, without empathy and without fear. It was as though 'He' was pointing at me and saying, 'This is what I can do, are you ready?'

Unbeknown to anyone, Mr C would return some years later to continue 'His' unfinished business. Again 'He' would quickly spin his web, taking Jean's loving husband, John away, closely followed by Eve, Jean's mother. Like Jean, both were just normal, everyday people, like you and me.

The weekend passed with all the sadness and solemness I'm sure you, the reader, can understand. Memories and tears were plentiful. Briefly, the good memories produced smiles and some laughter but were overwhelmed by pain and grief.

My appointment with Professor Shamari was nearing and, of course, I was apprehensive, but, now things could not come quickly enough. I was becoming easily fatigued, passing blood at least ten times a day and suffering from the stomach cramps. My meeting with the Professor was only a very small step on my journey but, as we all know, the longest journeys begin with those first, tentative steps.

I drove to the hospital alone. I wanted it that way. I was about to meet with someone I had never met and tell him what I had been suffering, in intimate details. I didn't, necessarily, want my loved ones to hear what suffering I had undergone during the last four months or so. It was my choice.

Having parked my car in the small car park to the front of the building, I waited as I was a few minutes early. I could see the hospital, a brick building, made up of two storeys. It was set in its own grounds, with trees and bushes hiding it from the main road. A narrow, winding driveway, dotted with speed humps, led from the main road to the hospital car park. From my parked position I could see the entrance into the main building, an automatic sliding door, situated at the bottom of a small flight of concrete steps. A small, narrow path led from my parked position to this entrance. Next to the steps was a ramp, presumably for wheelchair users and those who were unable to ascend or descend the steps, for whatever reasons.

As I waited, a number of people entered and exited the main entrance. Some were elderly, some not. Some walked freely, others did not. I then saw something completely unexpected. A peacock, in all its colourful glory, walked from right to left, immediately in front of my car. It was in no rush, just going about its business as it walked away, disappearing from sight, into the undergrowth. Seeing this majestic creature calmed me somewhat and I could almost feel my heartbeat slowing as I watched it peacefully disappear.

'You don't get that on the NHS!' I thought to myself.

As I walked down the steps towards the entrance, the automatic doors worked perfectly and I entered the hospital. I could see the reception desk, approximately thirty metres ahead of me, manned by three receptionists, busily typing away at their computers. There were seats aligned against each side wall, facing each other, and the walkway towards the reception area ran between them. As I approached, one of the receptionists raised her head. She politely enquired how she could help me and I explained the purpose of my visit to her. She asked me to hand over my credit card, which I did, and its details were taken. I was then asked to fill out a brief form, which included the details of my insurers, the authorisation code and the account number they had supplied me with. I was then invited to have a seat in the waiting area.

I noted there was a coffee machine and a vending machine close by. There were two corridors, one to the left and one to the right, leading away from the waiting area, deeper into the hospital.

I sat patiently, nervously waiting for my name to be called. I used the toilet which was close by, cleaning myself, before returning to my seat.

A gentleman then appeared from the right hand corridor. He was of western Asian appearance with dark, thinning hair and around my age. He was well-dressed in light-coloured trousers, black shiny shoes and a formal shirt. He stopped some three metres from me and called out my name. I rose and as I approached, he introduced himself as Professor Shamari.

I followed him along the right-hand corridor and we entered a small office. He sat down at a desk and he invited me to sit opposite him. After a few pleasantries, I explained to him the extent of the problems I had been suffering. He had a good sense of humour, putting me immediately at ease. I recall telling him that I was visiting the toilet at least ten times a day to empty my bowels, mainly passing blood. He was quite at ease with the information I was giving him.

'You won't need an enema then!' he jovially replied, a wry smile on his face.

The Professor then checked his schedule. He said he would make an appointment for me to undergo a sigmoidoscopy and explained the procedure to me. He made the appointment for the coming Thursday at 17:00, however, I should arrive at the hospital at 12:00. I would be shown to my own private room where I would wait. We then said our farewells and I left.

It seemed to me that my attendance at the hospital had taken at least an hour. Upon checking my watch, just fifteen minutes had passed.

There were no significant changes to my body over the next few days. My wife continued mourning the loss of her mother, with the family rallying around her. Her sister, who lived around an hour's drive away, would stay at either her father's house or ours. I would often see my wife pretending to watch the television but, in reality, she wasn't. Her mind wandered as she stared vacantly ahead. This would last several minutes before her tears began to flow. I comforted her as best I could, but I knew my efforts were weak and often seemed meaningless. After all, I could not take away the pain of her mother's loss. It was not just the loss of Jean, but the way she had been taken. The merciless way the cancer had 'eaten' away at her body and mind, reducing her to a shell of her former self.

My own journey was just beginning. At the moment the steps I was taking were small, but at least I was now walking in the right direction. I had no idea where it would lead but I knew it would be a difficult one. One aspect of my journey was in no doubt: that it would take me to places I had never thought I would go and certainly would never wish to.

CHAPTER THREE

Let the Air Out!

On Thursday 7th April 2016 at 12:00, I attended the hospital to undergo my sigmoidoscopy. I was shown to a private room on the first floor. It was an airy room, well-lit by the spring sunshine which penetrated the room through the large window at the rear of the room. It was furnished with a bed, and a television which sat upon a desk. Two chairs stood at each end of the desk. The room had an en suite bathroom attached to it, housing a sink, toilet and bath, including a shower.

The nurse who led me to the room stated that in a few hours someone would visit me and an enema would be carried out. I immediately had visions of a nurse similar to a Hattie Jacques type character from the 'Carry On Films' attending to me, being direct and manhandling me into the dreaded position. I smiled to myself, somewhat nervously. The nurse told me that at around 15:00 I should undress and put on the obligatory hospital gown. I'm sure you know the type: it's the back-to-front type with the ties at the back, which you can never do up properly!

The nurse left and I was alone. I stared out of the large window for several minutes, taking in the view of the neatly presented lawns and the rows of large trees which surrounded the bricked buildings. From the window I spied the resident peacock once more meandering on the lawn, just going about his or her business, before disappearing into the tree line.

I waited impatiently. The minutes ticked by slowly. I watched some daytime television which, as a lot of people know, is somewhat repetitive and did not aid the speeding of time. I visited the toilet regularly, passing my normal 'mixture'. As the clock approached 15:00, I undressed, placing my clothes neatly on one of the chairs. After numerous attempts, I managed to don the gown securely around my body, although I realised that any sudden movements and the ties would undo and I would be back, attempting to tie a secure knot once more.

Peculiar as it may seem, despite my nervousness, there was nowhere else I'd rather have been. You see, I was, hopefully, about to get a real insight into what had been causing me so much pain, fatigue, anxiety and fear for such a long time now. Finally, after the minutes, hours and days of the last four months, I felt I was getting somewhere. I knew this was only the beginning, but I also knew that without any knowledge of my enemy, it couldn't be fought. I was completely blind to what was occurring within my body but, now, with some luck, I would gain some insight upon my foe and be able to battle against it.

Around 15:30 there was a knock at the door.

'Come in,' I said, instinctively.

The door opened inwards and there stood my nurse,

'Hattie', only her appearance was nothing like the Hattie I had imagined. She was approximately five feet eight inches tall and of slim build. She had long straight fair hair and was around twenty-five years old. Her nurse's uniform almost fitted her physique perfectly, showing off her feminine lines. She was definitely no "Hattie" and reminded me more of Elle Macpherson. My heart sank. I would much rather have had Hattie attending to me than the Elle Macpherson of the nursing world. Why? Pure embarrassment, I'm afraid.

'Elle' entered the room and I could see she was holding something in her right hand. It resembled what, to me, looked like a baby's bottle but the 'teat' was clearly longer, thinner and, disconcertingly, much firmer. The 'teat' was about four inches in length and shaped like a very thin triangle with the point at the top.

She introduced herself as Louise and, without taking a breath, told me she had come for my enema.

'No problem, give it here and I'll do it,' I replied naively.

'No,' 'Elle' replied. 'I've got to do it!'

My heart sank even further. She invited me to undo my gown and lay on the bed on my left side, which I did. She then asked me to keep my legs together and raise my knees towards my chest. She parted my gown further and told me to keep still. I felt my heart rate rising rapidly and she began her task. I felt the liquid entering my body as she squeezed the 'baby's bottle', fully emptying its contents into me.

Again, there was no pain, just a mild discomfort. The

experience lasted seconds and the thought of what was going to occur was much worse than the reality. As 'Elle' removed her blue latex gloves, she explained I needed to wait at least five to ten minutes to allow for the optimum effect of the liquid she had squirted into me. I agreed that I would do my best as she walked away from me, towards the door to my room. As she opened it, she said goodbye.

'It was lovely to meet you!' I replied.

She smiled and closed the door behind her. I never saw 'Elle' again, our intimacy being very brief. I couldn't help thinking that some people would have paid good money for what I had just experienced!

Almost as soon as 'Elle' had closed the door, I felt the 'urge.' I held on to this urge for as long as I could, which was more like thirty seconds as opposed to five minutes, and found myself dashing into the bathroom to release the liquid which had so recently been forced into my body. I returned to my bed and as I waited impatiently, varying thoughts ran ever more rapidly through my mind. The time for my camera action was becoming ever closer and I could only imagine what that entailed. Would it cause pain? I had no idea, having never undergone such a procedure. Would it cause embarrassment? Undoubtedly. What would be discovered? I had no idea but whatever it was would not be pleasant.

At around 16:45 there was a further knock at my door. A nurse entered. She was neither 'Hattie' nor 'Elle'. She explained that the time for my sigmoidoscopy had arrived and led me from my room along a short corridor where empty mobile hospital beds were pushed against one side. The ties on my gown, thankfully, remained in place and I followed the nurse into a small room at the end of the corridor.

In this room was another nurse and a face I recognised: Professor Shamari. He greeted me, attempting to put me at ease. Despite his attempts, my fears remained. Within the room was a mobile hospital bed along with various medical 'machinery.' I noted that on one side of the bed was a large television screen facing the bed. Not more daytime television, please! In a way it actually would be, with me, or at least parts of me, being the star of the show!

A nurse invited me to lie on the bed and to roll onto my left side. I undid the ties that held my gown in its position. The TV screen was directly in my eye-line and was clearly switched on, although the screen remained blank. I was asked to raise my knees towards my chest, which I did. Both nurses were wearing surgical masks and gloves along with their blue surgical gowns. Professor Shamari was also donned in a similar outfit and he moved out of sight behind me.

I felt a cool, moist sensation between each buttock and realised that some sort of gel had been applied. The screen in front of me now sprang into life. My buttocks and anus were now visible on the large, flat screen and as the camera was moved nearer, the picture became much clearer. As the camera entered my body, I felt myself tensing and was told to relax and keep still by the Professor. Keeping still wasn't a problem but relaxing definitely was! As the camera was pushed into my body, there was no pain, just the mild discomfort I was now accustomed to. I relaxed a little. The light on the end of the camera lit up my insides as it made its way into my lower bowel. All was displayed on the screen to me and the Professor. I watched, amazed as the minute camera, followed by the even smaller lead which powered it, was pushed deeper inside me. It was, literally, like the smallest tunnelling machine you could ever imagine. Deeper it went, its path being cleared by jets of air being propelled from the front of the camera. Attached to the side of the camera I could see what looked like the gripping part of a tiny pair of pliers. As the air entered my body, I very quickly felt the urge to pass wind. Since the Professor was positioned directly behind me, I resisted the urge. However, with each split second that passed, the urge became stronger. As I resisted, I felt a sharp pain inside me and my body visibly tensed. The pain became more intense, the type of pain which begins to take over, taking your breath away.

The Professor immediately realised what was happening and in no uncertain terms exclaimed, "Let the air out! Now!"

By now the camera had only been inside me for a matter of seconds and I was holding in the air, primarily to protect the camera operator from being sprayed by the air which had built up inside me and whatever material was mixed with that air. At this stage, that was my only thought. But the few words the Professor had spoken were enough and as soon as they left his lips, I immediately relaxed. The air was expelled from my anus. It seemed to be one lasting rush of air and whatever else, leaving my very soul. The whole time, the camera and its attachments continued on their journey, the air continually clearing a path and making the camera view clear. No sooner had the air jetted forward than it seemed to reverse its forward momentum and was expelled from where the camera had originally entered.

I had terrible visions of the poor Professor being pelted by whatever material was being propelled from my body as the air rushed from me, unfortunately in his direction. I prayed he was wearing adequate personal protective equipment!

As I expelled the air, in what seemed one continuous motion, the pain left my body as quickly as it had arrived. I now experienced no pain as the expulsion continued and the camera meandered its way deeper into my lower bowel. The tiny torch lit its way and the air cleared its path.

I was completely amazed by what I was seeing on the big screen, all in high definition. The very inner workings of my body were being displayed in all their glory and, as I had imagined, my bowel resembled a very narrow tunnel.

Then, as if by magic, there it was! Professor Shamari brought the camera to an abrupt halt. The torch shone on the 'culprit' which had been causing all my problems over the previous months. The 'spectre' of my insides which had caused such anguish, uncertainty, pain, fear and embarrassment, the numerous toilet visits and the physical and mental weakening, was displayed in all its infamous glory on the screen directly in front of my eyes. We had now, literally, come face to face.

The camera had revealed a growth in my lower bowel. It was shaped like a tiny human thumb and protruded from the right side of my lower bowel toward the left side. It had grown horizontally, approximately three quarters of the way across my bowel. There was a small gap between it and the top and bottom walls of the 'tunnel', which made up my lower bowel. The end of the growth, which had not quite reached the left wall, was much darker in colour to the rest of it, almost black. It reminded me of a stalactite in an oval-shaped cave, increasing from a small growth into a large one, almost touching the ground below it, but this particular stalactite had grown, and was still growing, horizontally from right to left.

The Professor now spoke.

'You may feel a little discomfort.'

I didn't reply. As he finished speaking, the camera was pushed forward a little and the mouth of the 'plier-like' attachment opened like a baby bird's beak opens when its mother returns with a fresh meal. The 'pliers' then shut forcibly on a small part of the growth, before the camera and its attachments moved slowly backwards. A few small specks of blood discharged themselves, appearing to float as if in air, as a part of the growth was cut away and held in the jaws of the 'pliers'. The camera, complete with its attachments, began reversing and a second later they smoothly exited my body.

Remaining in my position, I managed to utter a few words

from my now very dry lips.

'What do you think it is?' I asked, immediately realising the stupidity of the words I had spoken. Both Professor Shamari and I knew exactly what it was. He need not have replied but he did.

'I think it's cancer,' he said clearly. He explained to me that my 'growth' was too large for him to remove with the equipment attached to the camera. He took a mobile telephone from one of his pockets and stated he was going to phone Mr Syed, one of the surgeons at the hospital. He did so but there was no reply.

He told me that a biopsy had been taken and the hospital would be in contact to arrange a Computerised Tomography (CT) scan, which would take place in the very near future. The nurse then led me back to my room, where I dressed myself, left the hospital and drove home, still trying to comprehend what I had seen inside my body. Although my attendance at the hospital had lasted around five and a half hours, the procedure I had undergone had only lasted approximately ten minutes.

Arriving home, I explained to my wife, as best I could, what had been seen within me. We hugged and she offered words of comfort to me. Although nothing had yet been confirmed, I didn't need to tell her that my 'growth' was a tumour caused by cancer. It was very obvious to me and would have been to anyone who saw it. My son and I had a brief conversation and although shocked, he offered words of comfort and love. My wife telephoned our daughter to explain my situation to her. Words were brief between them. It was what it was and there was nothing we could do about it. We couldn't pretend it wasn't there and we were unable to turn back time, to alter what had occurred. The only thing now was the future and how to deal with it.

That night, I woke several times. My mind was racing but I was actually looking forward to the future. I would take each day as it came, despite having little idea of the procedures I would be facing. I looked forward to the day I would be healthy again, although I had no idea when that would be. I had no experience of being seriously ill and these were the early steps of my journey. You never know when illness will strike. There is no date pencilled in on the calendar to warn you. We all know that's not how it works. Although I knew and had heard of people suffering from cancer, I never thought it would happen to me. I had never entertained the thought of being diagnosed with cancer. Why should it be me? The question I should have asked myself was, 'Why shouldn't it be me?' After all I'm no different to you or the majority of the human population. We are all really the same. Anyone asking, 'Why me?' should really be asking the question, 'Why not me?'

CHAPTER FOUR

Judgement Day and Some Barium and Iodine

The following day, I went to work as normal. I explained to my work colleagues there was a possibility I had cancer, although nothing had been confirmed, and I was awaiting biopsy results. Again comforting and supportive words filled the air, as you would expect. The possibility that I had cancer did not change their lives. I was not their priority. Just like me, they had families and their own lives to contend with and we all know the challenges this can present.

I continued my daily work. My toilet visits were the same in quantity and quality. The same 'material' left my body. It didn't really change in this short period since my camera experience. I did my best to remain upbeat, whilst also being worried about what the future held in store for me. I was looking forward to the day my horizontal stalactite would be taken from me, freeing me again. I wished and longed for the day when I would undergo whatever procedure was required.

Several days later, I received correspondence from the hospital. An appointment had been made for me to undergo a CT scan. Again, this was to be a new experience for me and I had very little knowledge of what to expect. The day after the scan I would have a consultation with the surgeon, Mr Syed, the gentleman whom Professor Shamari had attempted to contact following my sigmoidoscopy. My scan was to take place during the afternoon of 18th April 2016. Both appointments would take place at the private hospital and I could not wait! I was like a child, waking during the early hours of Christmas Day, unable to sleep due to the expectancy of what would soon be theirs. The ball was properly rolling now and with each day that passed it gained a little in speed. I hoped beyond hope nothing would slow its progress.

During the afternoon of 18th April 2016, I drove from my home address to the hospital, my wife beside me. The journey was a short one, only taking fifteen minutes or so. As I entered the grounds of the hospital, which was unfortunately built next to the local crematorium, I admired the large trees aligning the meandering, narrow, road which led to the hospital car park. I parked my car, and my wife and I entered the hospital. We walked through the main waiting area, turning left at reception, and made our way along a narrow corridor. We then turned left again into the waiting area of the X-ray and scanning department. A brief conversation took place with the receptionist and we both sat quietly on the chairs provided, as if we were children waiting to be called into the headmaster's office. A few minutes later, the door opened and we were invited into the department, where, once more, we sat. The room was small with doors leading to various other rooms and another corridor ran to our left. A nurse approached several minutes later, carrying a transparent plastic container which had liquid in it. It resembled a protein mixer bottle, the type you would use to mix a protein shake after visiting the gymnasium. The nurse placed the plastic bottle on a small, round table to my left-hand side. She then asked me to enter a small changing cubicle nearby, where I would find one of the dreaded back-to-front gowns along with a pair of disposable slippers. She asked me to change, which I did, making sure I also removed any jewellery I was wearing with the exception of my wedding ring. When I returned, she explained that I needed to drink the liquid in the container. I was told I should drink it in small doses, making sure it had all been consumed, over the next hour. I enquired what the liquid was and she explained that the container was filled with a substance called barium. Once consumed, the barium would help give a clearer view of my organs whilst I was undergoing my scan.

I began to drink the barium, continuing to do so over the next hour. The liquid was white in colour, having the texture of a very watered-down milkshake. Over the next hour, although the taste was unpleasant, I managed to drink the full amount, approximately one litre. Within minutes of finishing the excuse of a milkshake, the nurse approached and I was led to the scanning room.

A cannula was inserted into the main vein on top of my right hand and it was explained that the purpose of this was so that an iodinated contrast, basically iodine, could be injected into me, again helping with the 'viewing' process. The nurse also told me that once the contrast was injected, I would feel as though I had lost control of my bladder and would feel like I had wet myself. She told me that in all her years of experience she'd only ever known one person, an elderly gentleman, actually wet themself. Inwardly I prayed I would not be number two!

The nurse explained that although she wouldn't be in the room with me when the scanning commenced, she would be able to see me from her position and would speak to me via an intercom which was incorporated into the scanner. She would tell me when I was to hold my breath and when to release it. Whilst holding my breath, I would be still and the scanning would take place.

The machine was exactly how you'd imagine it to be. It was like a large ring which would pass over my body, stopping in the correct position over my torso, with my legs, feet and head protruding from it.

Having removed my gown, I lay on the bed which then entered the scanner, stopping when in the correct position. 'Let the scanning commence!' I thought to myself as the machine whirred into life. I held and released my breath when instructed to do so by the nurse, so the radiographer who accompanied her in a small office, within the scanning room, could complete his work.

After several minutes of holding and releasing my breath, the nurse left the protected room and injected the iodine mixture into my cannula. Her explanation regarding the effects of the iodine was inaccurate in one small detail: within a split second of the fluid entering my bloodstream, I felt the front of my underwear warming, convincing me I had wet myself. Not only did the front of my underwear begin to warm, so did the back! The feeling was so real that I was convinced I had not only wet myself, but also soiled myself. I found myself recalling the nurse's words and kept telling myself over and over that nothing, front nor back, had seeped from my prone body. It didn't work. No matter how many times her words ran through my brain I was utterly convinced that, once I left that bed, I would be leaving a huge mess in my wake.

A few more minutes passed and the nurse spoke to me through the intercom inside the scanning machine, informing me that I could leave the bed and replace my gown.

Fear consumed me as I rose from the bed. My heart was thumping so loudly I could almost hear it. Immediately I looked to where I had been laying, expecting to see a complete mess. Nothing, not a thing. Not even a sweat mark! I glanced down at the front of my underwear and still nothing. My heart returned to its normal speed and my relief almost overwhelmed me.

I replaced my gown and the nurse removed my cannula. I thanked the nurse, left the room, changed and my wife and I left the hospital. I relayed my experiences to my wife, telling her that I could not believe I had not left a sodden mess behind in the scanning room. We chuckled together and returned home, awaiting the next day's instalment at the hospital and my appointment with Mr Syed.

The next day arrived just like any other day, but this was not just any other day. Whatever had been seen, whatever had been discovered inside my body, and whatever Mr Syed was going to say to me at our upcoming meeting, would change my life. Would I be told that the 'being' invading my lower bowel was also invading other parts of me? Had it spread? Would my liver, lungs or any other of my vital organs have been affected? Had it infiltrated my body to such an extent that any treatment would be futile? Surely not. I felt like I had become the guilty man in the dock, awaiting judgement. What would my sentence be? Would I become the condemned man? What would happen to my family, friends and loved ones if that was the case? These thoughts were pushed from my mind and locked out. The thought of dying had not really entered my mind, not since my problems began, not through my initial meetings and appointments. No way was I about to start entertaining any thoughts of 'shuffling off this mortal coil.' No way was my parasite going to cause that. NO WAY!

On the 19th April 2016, at around 19:00, I attended the hospital, my wife with me, and booked in at reception. The receptionist, a lady in her mid-twenties, told me Mr Syed was running late but she hoped I wasn't going to be kept waiting too long. I took a seat in the waiting room next to my wife who was already seated. Several people of varying ages and descriptions filled the majority of the seats. For some unknown and ignorant reason, I had always envisaged only the more 'well-off' would be sitting in the waiting room of a private hospital. I had expected to see men in suits with well-polished shoes and ladies in expensive, smart dresses and clutching at designer handbags filling the room, looking down their noses at 'normal' me. This wasn't the case. Yes, it's true to say that there were a few of these types patiently waiting, but the vast majority of them were just like me. There were parents whose small children caused havoc as they ran amok, slim people, overweight people, scruffy people, smart people, people using crutches and those who moved freely. There were noisy people, you know the type, those who want everyone to hear their conversations, and those who remained silent, just staring blankly ahead. Without the comfy seats and vending machines, it could have passed for any surgery waiting room.

Various professional looking people walked from the corridors either side of reception with an almost perfect frequency. These professionals would stop in front of reception and call out the names of their next patients. The actual doctors and consultants performed the name calling, something I had not experienced prior to this visit. It seemed all very informal. Perhaps this was how it was supposed to be, putting the patient's minds at rest, prior to giving them their news.

Having had their names called, the patients would rise nervously from their seats and follow their chosen professionals along the corridor and out of sight, only to return a short while later.

My wife and I both waited patiently. The minutes ticked by and as they did so, my patience began to wane. I so wanted my meeting with 'my professional' and so wanted to hear the news, however bad that news was. I imagined Mr Syed appearing, as if in a puff of smoke, and calling my name. No puff of smoke appeared, the minutes ticked by and it seemed, by now, I was examining my watch by the minute.

I visited the toilet to make sure everything was in order before returning to my seat, muttering, almost inaudibly, to my wife.

'Where is he then?'

Although my question was not meant to be rhetorical, no reply was forthcoming. The wait continued, me checking my watch. I wanted to be put out of my misery, to have my diagnosis confirmed.

As my watch ticked over to 20:15, the automatic doors at the hospital entrance opened, with the uniform sound these machines make. A male entered. He was smartly dressed in light-coloured trousers and a darker buttoned-up shirt. He was around ten years my junior, approximately six feet tall and of slim build. He was of Indian appearance with neatly trimmed, black hair, sporting grey flecks to the sides. Instantly, I knew who he was. He strode purposefully along the narrow walkway, aligned by patients comfortably sitting in their individual seats. As he got closer, I noted he had the most stunning eyes. They were not dark as you would imagine, but a light to mid grey, and piercing. Against his dark features they stood out like beacons of light on a black night. He looked familiar to me, although I did not know why this was the case. Somehow, I knew him. Somehow, I was convinced our paths had previously crossed but I could not place where or when.

He continued, passing my position, turning right along the corridor and disappeared from view.

'That's him,' I informed my wife.

'Could be,' she retorted, continuing to stare at the pages of a magazine which, by now, had clearly engulfed her.

Both my saviour and executioner had arrived at once, in the form of Mr Syed.

A few minutes later he returned, standing next to the reception desk, scanning the waiting room.

I began to ready myself, rising very slightly from my seated position, when I heard him call out, 'Mr Jones, please.'

Mr Jones and Mr Syed then disappeared along the corridor. My wife looked up from the pages she had been concentrating on and commented, 'We know what Mr Jones is here for, don't we?'

Our eyes met and a guarded smile parted our lips.

Some twenty minutes later, Mr Jones re-appeared. He walked past me, through the automatic doors and away into the night. Time now ticked more slowly than ever, each minute passing as though it was an hour, before 'Smoky Eyes' appeared once more, saying the words I had longed for: 'Mr Michaels, please.'

My wife and I stood as one and Mr Syed nodded his

acknowledgement in my direction, before turning and heading along the corridor. We both followed and a few steps into the corridor, he opened a door to an office on the right-hand side, politely inviting us in. He offered each of us a seat and sat opposite us at his desk. He introduced himself, apologised for his lateness, explaining that he had been delayed as he was urgently operating on a gentleman who was suffering from bowel cancer. Immediately, an image of an elderly man lying unconscious on a hospital bed entered my mind. Mr Syed immediately took those thoughts away. He explained that this patient was only thirty years old and my thoughts immediately went out to this poor individual. Thirty years old! My ignorance had influenced my thoughts, making them inaccurate almost beyond belief.

Immediately, I felt guilty about my impatience and assured Mr Syed that no apology was necessary. He began thumbing through a file of papers on his desk, studying them intently. I stared blankly in his direction, trying to read his thoughts. After a few, very long moments, he looked up.

'I can confirm it is cancer.' His words were blunt, but what else could they be? Did my world collapse with his words? Did I think my sentence was terminal? Did I break down? No, I did not. Although shocked, I was not surprised. I had seen, in high definition, what was invading my lower bowel and these words were expected. I said nothing and nor did my wife. An awkward silence filled the room. 'Smoky Eyes' continued.

'You will need an operation, which I will perform.'

He began scribbling on a piece of paper lying on the desk in front of him, drawing a picture which allowed him to explain to us where the tumour was in my body. He informed us that had the cancer grown in a slightly lower position, the operation would have been much more complicated, being closer to my anus, and making surgery much more difficult. I didn't speak, just listened. He continued saying that as I was relatively young and fit, he expected me to make a full recovery and lead a full and healthy life. He further explained that, following surgery, I would probably need to spend about five days in hospital and then six to eight weeks recuperating at home. He told me that there was a possibility that I may need to be fitted with a stoma (colostomy bag) which I would need to wear either temporarily or permanently. He hoped this wouldn't be the case but would not know until my procedure was carried out. To me, this was a small price to pay for the removal of my invader and the end of my pain, anguish and fears.

Mr Syed dispelled my greatest fear with his next words. He reassured me that the cancer had not spread to any of my other organs. This was something that had troubled me throughout the last months. Had it been the case that other vital organs had been affected, I would probably have felt somewhat doomed, but he reassured me this was not the case. When he did so, I exhaled audibly, a sense of relief overwhelming me. The beast within me had been imprisoned in my bowel and had not escaped, making its execution so much easier.

'Smoky Eyes' explained further: during my surgery, a number of incisions would be made into my stomach area, robotically. These would be performed by what was known as a 'da Vinci Robot' which would be operated by him as he sat nearby at a monitor. This was a relatively new method but made the surgeon's task less complicated and meant recovery times were reduced.

The operation would not take place at the private hospital, but in the local general hospital, close by. Prior to my operation, I would need to undergo a Magnetic Resonance Imaging (MRI) scan, which would give an even clearer picture of my insides and exactly where my invader was.

I listened intently, trying to understand all that Mr Syed was telling me. This was brand new to me, and new experiences were heading toward me, racing my way, and I couldn't wait for them to arrive. My underlying thought was that I wanted rid of what was growing inside me, and the quicker, the better. If 'Smoky Eyes' had said to me he was able to perform the operation the next day, I would have probably jumped from my seat, vaulted the desk and kissed him, passionately! Luckily for him he didn't!

Once he had explained to me the procedures I would have to undergo, I began to feel more at ease. I knew my immediate future was going to be hard going, with pain and anguish along the way, but I looked beyond that, to when I wouldn't be constantly visiting the lavatory, not having to clean myself at regular intervals, not suffering the stomach cramps, not being constantly fatigued and, overwhelmingly, worrying about what was occurring inside my body.

'Smoky Eyes' naturally asked me if I had any questions. Obviously, I had tried to take in all that he had told me, but I found any questions difficult to find as my brain began processing the information it had just received. I couldn't think of anything to ask him, other than how quickly the operation would or could take place. He was unable to answer this question, assuring me it would be done as soon as was possible.

My next response clearly put him on his back foot.

'I'm sure I know you from somewhere,' I said quizzically.

I could feel my wife's eyes burning into the side of my head; her disbelieving silence was eminent. Before he could reply, it came to me.

'Cricket!' I proclaimed proudly.

I recalled that one sunny Saturday afternoon the previous summer I was involved in a local cup game. The opposition were a player short when the game began, but the player who was late arrived some twenty minutes after play began, running hurriedly and apologetically onto the field of play. He seemed just a normal guy, late for an amateur game, not an unusual occurrence. What was unusual was the reason he was late. I heard the opposing captain explaining to a teammate that 'Mr Late' was a surgeon at the hospital nearby and had been working that morning. It was not uncommon for him to be late as often his work took longer than planned and it was not something he could stop mid flow, returning to complete his task at a later date.

I also recalled that during this particular match I had batted the best I had all season, scoring ninety-nine runs not out. We knocked 'Mr Late's' team out of the cup and I won the player of the match award. I relayed this to 'Smoky Eyes' and a peculiar bond immediately formed between us. It then occurred to me that maybe I shouldn't have reminded him that I had, almost single handily, knocked his beloved cricket team out of the cup. I really needn't have worried.

Mr Syed remembered the game well. We spoke for a few minutes about our joint love of cricket, before saying our farewells. My wife and I left the hospital, still trying to comprehend what the consultant had relayed to us.

It may sound peculiar to say this, but I didn't feel downcast by what I had been told. I felt hope for the future and that it was now assured. I would have the operation and then all would be well. All I needed to do was get through my surgery, recover and begin living my life as normal. Unfortunately, nature had other plans for me. More pain, more anguish and more uncertainty. I just didn't know it yet.

I drove away from the hospital, almost rejoicing. I remember saying to my wife that although I had cancer, I was happy. That may sound very odd but you must understand that having cancer didn't make me happy. I'm not a fool, but now it was not the unknown I was fighting. I knew where it was, what it was and with these discoveries it could be fought and, hopefully, defeated. The invader had changed my life over these past months but now I felt the tables had begun to turn. Whereas the cancer within me had confused, frightened and consumed my thoughts almost every second of each day, using its weapons against me, I now had my own formidable weapon to fight back with, in the form of Mr Syed.

Leaving the hospital on that pleasant, spring evening I decided to visit my parents. I had not informed them of any of my problems. They did not see me daily, so I was able to keep my suffering from them. My wife, son, daughter and work colleagues saw me almost every day, so I saw fit to furnish them with some details of what I was experiencing. To them, my diagnosis, although sad, would not be a shock. My parents had no snippets of information, so what I was about to tell them was going to be completely out of the blue. I knew it would shock them to their cores, but it was something I was unable to protect them from any longer. I had dwelled on the idea of telling them but I decided that if my son were in my position, I would want to know.

My wife and I entered my parent's property. The front door to their bungalow was unlocked, even though it was past nine o'clock. I had often asked them to keep their door locked. However, like many people in their eighties, they had their routine and no matter how many times I asked, their routine was primary.

I hurried into the large living room before any sounds of our impending arrival could alert them. We were greeted by them but, due to the late hour of our visit, they instinctively knew something was not right.

Both of us sat down and were offered drinks which we declined. With my mother and father sitting opposite, I began. I could not pussyfoot around and I told them I had some bad news, explaining that I had just come from the hospital where it had been confirmed that I had cancer. Plans were underway for me to undergo an operation and I had been told by the experts that all was expected to work out well.

Naturally, both were extremely shocked and stunned at my news. They sat silently processing the information I had just delivered. My mother rose and I followed her lead. We embraced. No words were spoken and none were needed. I continued re-assuring them that I would be fine. No tears flowed, although their faces were full of sadness. Their youngest son, the boy they had nurtured through childhood and adolescence into manhood had just given them the terrible news that he was suffering a life-threatening illness.

Words were few between us. The shock was obvious and the sadness plain to see. I was saddened to have to break this news to them but felt better now I had. It would have been unfair to have kept it from them any longer. It was what it was. My re-assurances continued and I told them that after my operation I would be fine and make a full recovery. The invader would be removed and that would be it. A few weeks later, I would be back to full fitness and continuing as normal.

When the time came for us to leave, hugs were exchanged. Words were still hard to find. What else could I tell them? I couldn't tell them anymore as I didn't know anymore. They knew as much as I knew.

Driving home, it occurred to me that I had just experienced one of the most difficult things I had ever had to do. I wanted to protect my elderly parents as much as I could and had done so up to this point, but now my invader had reached out its tentacles like an octopus wraps its prey and pulled my parents into its cancerous world. As time passed, more and more people, people who were dear to me, were becoming entangled in its sprawling and unforgiving web. It was reaching out in ever-increasing circles, punishing not just those whom it had invaded.

Back at home, both our children were also told that my cancer was now confirmed. It was what they had expected and was not shocking to them, as it hadn't been to me. They had been forewarned by my wife and me and, as such, were forearmed. My wife telephoned her sister and brother to give them the news and I telephoned my brother. All were expecting what we were confirming, but it didn't lessen the hardship of telling them. In a way, telling those you love and are dear to you is worse than being diagnosed.

I dare say my sleep that night was deeper and sounder than that of my dear parents.

CHAPTER FIVE

Shoes and Enemas!

The following day I worked as usual, arriving at the office around 08:15. I immediately explained my diagnosis to my boss and the others who were present and words of support emanated from their lips. I was waiting for my friend, Patrick, who duly arrived just before 0900.

I was dressed in my usual attire of smart trousers and shirt; however, just one item was different. I had recently purchased a new pair of shoes. They were a shiny black leather, almost like a patent dress shoe, and this was their first outing. They were comfortable, good quality and made from Italian leather. I knew that Patrick, a person who liked fashionable items and always dressed smartly, would approve.

As we spoke, I told him it was now official. I had been diagnosed and would soon be operated upon. We embraced, patting each other on the back, as men in these situations often do. He offered me words of comfort and support. As we spoke, his eyes averted down to my shiny Italian leather shoes. He paused momentarily and whilst still staring at my shoes, said, 'They're nice shoes.'

Before I could reply, he continued with the question, 'What size shoe are you?'

He looked at me and I at him. We both smiled, our smiles becoming wider until we were both laughing out loud. I knew he meant what he was saying as a joke and he knew I'd take it that way, which I did. Should my illness have taken its ultimate prize, I would have made sure that on the morning of my passing, those shoes would have been placed in the centre of his desk before 09:00, to greet him upon his arrival. I also knew that the placing of my shoes would not be necessary.

The following day was another sad one. The day of lovely Jean's cremation had arrived. As far as these things can do, it went 'well'. Numerous people were in attendance, her family and friends. Some I recognised, some I did not. John, Jean's ever-loving husband, had planned a small speech, a final goodbye to his love, as the coffin was in situ. When the time arrived, he was unable to deliver his words. Emotions overwhelmed him, robbing him of the words he longed to say. In any other setting it would have been an awkward moment but here it wasn't. Everybody knew of his devotion to his wonderful wife, of the years they had spent together, the good and not so good times. He returned to his seat, escorted by a close friend. Tears from the children, grandchildren and loved ones followed. Mr C had touched not only his beloved Jean but, indirectly, all those present. Again, 'He' had cast his web, reaching out, drawing others in. I found it so sad and extremely ironic that I too had been diagnosed just two days earlier. Again, I thought, 'His' web was growing, undeterred, not pausing to decide who to affect. Many have been cut down by this disease and the effects have rippled far and wide, leaving great sadness in their wake.

I felt so sorry for my lovely wife, her sister and her brother. They had lost their mother so cruelly. Friends and acquaintances had lost a good friend, but my deepest sorrow was for Jean's mother. Here she was at ninety years of age, struggling to cope with her loss. Her only daughter was gone, taken from her. Her pain must have been unimaginable. We could only offer her words but words seemed meaningless at this time. What a complete fucking bastard this cancer is!

It was during Jean's wake that my mobile telephone rang. I recognised the number instantly – it was the hospital. I answered the call very nervously.

'Hello, Anthony Michaels speaking.'

It was Mr Syed's secretary calling.

'Hello Mr Michaels. I just wanted to let you know that we have booked you in for your operation on 19th May,' she politely replied.

I remained silent, gathering my thoughts. I felt deflated. The date of my operation was still almost a month away. I would have to endure passing blood, toilet visits, stomach cramps and fatigue for even longer! I could envisage the parasite within me smiling, wryly.

My silence prompted the secretary to continue.

'Mr Syed is due to attend a course in the United States, which is why your operation cannot be performed sooner.'

I thanked the secretary for the information but was saddened by her words. I longed for my invader to be gone and now the person who was going to remove it was jetting off to the States!

The emotional rollercoaster was again at one of its many troughs. There had been many more troughs than peaks on this journey. Elation and sadness seemed to flow side by side and there was very little I could do about it. I could only wait for the cancer to be cut out of me and now it seemed that was still a long way away. It was now only 21ˢᵗ April 2016.

Each day that passed was much as the previous one had been. Countless toilet visits, countless times spent cleaning myself and endless worries. Worries for myself and worries for my loved ones. I knew that the longer Mr C was within me, the more 'He' would wear me down and the more damage 'He' could and, probably, would inflict. I felt myself becoming weaker physically and mentally as each day passed. However, there was still one thought that didn't enter my mind: the thought of dying. I am sure that had Mr C wanted to change those thoughts, 'He; could have. 'He' didn't.

Five days after Jean's cremation, I received another call from the hospital. I was asked to attend the X-ray department in two days to undergo an MRI scan. My hopes again rose. More investigations would take place, ultimately leading to the end of my 'sentence' and the removal of my tumour.

Two days later I attended the hospital as requested. I won't bore you with the details, save to say it was a similar set-up to my CT scan. Removal of jewellery and gown wearing was again required. Thankfully, barium was not consumed on this occasion and was not missed.

As I lay prone on my back at the mercy of the whirring machine, it was explained that this procedure would take approximately forty-five minutes, around three times as long as my CT scan. This would be a very noisy procedure and I may feel a sensation of movement within my body. They weren't wrong!

A metal plate was placed over my stomach. This plate was approximately twelve inches long and six inches wide and around an inch in thickness. This time, the machine was longer, but the hollow part was narrower. I was given some headphones through which a wide range of songs were playing, and the bed began its motorised journey into the machine. I felt slightly claustrophobic as it whirred into life – the inner walls of the machine were only inches from my face and body. I held and released my breath when instructed. Whilst being scanned, it felt like my insides were moving as the magnets performed as expected. With each scan, the movement inside me increased. By the time the last scan was in progress, I was sure there was a tiny Spaniard within me, shaking his maracas vigorously! It felt like parts of my insides were exchanging places with other parts as the machine noisily went about its business.

No iodine injection was carried out, thankfully, and no worries about messing myself occurred. It was a painless process, just as my CT scan had been, but a totally different experience. I would liken it to how you would think it would feel if you entered a very noisy teleportation machine, taking you to another place, piece by piece, shaking your insides before removing them bit by bit, then rearranging them correctly elsewhere. A quick blood test later and I was on my way once more.

Following my latest scan, events began to move rapidly. I liaised with my insurers who had asked where my operation was to take place and whether it would be performed robotically. I informed them that it would take place at the local general hospital, robotically, but no date had yet been set.

Over the following days I spoke with Mr Syed's secretary on a number of occasions, along with representatives of the insurers. A dispute had now arisen as to whether my operation would take place robotically or manually. Numerous telephone calls ensued. Basically, it boiled down to that old devil called money.

The insurers were authorised to pay up to £8500.00 for my operation but were told that the cost of using the da Vinci robot would cost around £10,500.00. Manually, the cost would be £8500.00. Again, I felt somewhat deflated. And again, my rollercoaster entered one of its troughs, not because of the invader within but because of money. My Syed's secretary confirmed that if the insurers were unmoved, the operation would still take place, but manually. She added that the consultant had contacted the insurers personally and had explained the benefits of performing the procedure via the robot, but his pleadings fell on deaf ears.

To me, it didn't really matter how the operation was performed but I was worried that the financial argument would delay the procedure. By now, if I had been tied down, a rag inserted into my mouth and someone had heated a large, sharp knife and started cutting into me, it would have been worth it just to be rid of my invader forever.

On the 4th May 2016, I received word that I was to undergo a pre-op investigation at the private suite in the general hospital. This was to take place the following day and Mr Syed was due back at work on 6th May, having returned from America early, Mr Syed's secretary continued, telling me the words I had longed to hear. My operation was to be carried out on Saturday 7th May 2016, three days from now! I was absolutely elated. My emotional rollercoaster was at a peak. By now it seemed to be a series of peaks and troughs, one rapidly following the other.

My pre-op went well, although my blood pressure was a little high. My blood pressure was a little high! I wasn't surprised, having struggled mentally and physically with so much during the past months. It came as no surprise but I felt nothing was going to stop me now. My invader had almost come to its grisly end and no tears were going to be shed upon its demise.

I was told I had to attend the Nelson Suite at the general hospital on the morning of 7th May at around 07:30. As it was to be a Saturday operation, I hoped that 'Smoky Eyes' was not playing cricket on that day! After all, I wanted his attention to be solely focused on my bowel and not on how many runs he would be scoring that afternoon. Again, I needn't have worried!

The night prior to my operation I slept surprisingly well. I woke a number of times, checking the digital clock next to me. My waking moments were due more to excitement than fear. Even through sleep, I was peaking on the emotional rollercoaster I was riding. Despite the fact that I was due to undergo quite a lengthy operation, with my skin, flesh, tissue and muscle being cut into, I had little fear. I suspect that loved ones and those dearest to me suffered more fear than I did. After all, I would be present throughout the proceedings, whereas they would be going about their daily business as best they could, doing what people do. My closest family would be checking their mobile telephones whilst they shopped or watched their televisions, waiting for any news. I would be present, receiving the news firsthand, knowing how I felt, what pain I was in, whereas they would be unsure, wondering when news would come and what that news would be. No doubt they would be worrying unduly. I would be there, in the moment, having some control. At times like these, the fears and anxieties of my dearest would be magnified. I couldn't help feeling that although I was the one undergoing surgery, their fears would be greater.

Around 06:00 I awoke, showered and prepared myself for the day ahead. It was now only hours until I would be free to live my life once more as it had been placed on hold for far too long now. I was not frightened, just experiencing a mixture of relief and excitement. My time had now come just as a child's time comes on a Christmas or birthday morning.

My wife and I left our house around 07:00, my wife driving the ten-minute journey to the hospital as I sat in the passenger seat, clutching the small holdall which contained my toiletries and a small amount of clothes which would be my only possessions over the following days.

We were shown to a private room where, once again, I donned the almost impossible gown and waited for a pre-op meeting with 'smoky eyes.' I watched the minutes tick by, all too slowly, until he arrived. He was confident and professional, and I felt little concern for my wellbeing. After some pleasantries, he explained that, prior to me being taken to theatre, I would undergo two enemas to make sure my bowel was clean. I would then be escorted to theatre where he would undertake the operation manually. Before he left, we shook hands and, once again, I was peaking.

A few short minutes later, a nurse arrived, dressed in a dark blue overall. He introduced himself as Carlos and explained he was there to perform my first enema. He was a young man, in his early twenties, with short black hair, and of Mediterranean appearance. I knew what was about to occur as, from a pocket of his well-presented overall, he produced the small bottle with its triangle shaped lid. I assumed the position, not worried at all. After all, my previous experience of this position had caused only a little discomfort. Why should it be any different this time?

Unfortunately, it was. This was completely different. Lying on my right-hand side, my knees bent and my legs pulled towards my chest, I felt a very sharp, stabbing pain, directly above my anus. I yelled out in pain, looking wide-eyed and directly into my wife's eyes. The pain was excruciating and I could not control the emotion leaving my voice box and, subsequently, my lips. The pain left me as Carlos, clearly not finding his target, ceased his actions briefly before he made a further attempt. He missed again and the pain surged through me once more. It was as though he was trying to force the triangular point into a hole that wasn't there. He withdrew once more, all too briefly, before a further attempt was made. I could feel the point missing its target and I felt like I was being stabbed directly above my anus. I stared into my wife's eyes and she stared into mine. She could clearly see the agony I was in; her lips parted, as if to speak, as the triangular point eventually found its target and the contents of the bottle were squeezed into me.

The pain left my body as quickly as it had arrived. Carlos clearly knew that something was very wrong. He apologised to me for causing such pain, stating that he 'must have hit a pile' as he sheepishly left the room.

I immediately left the bed and entered the en suite bathroom. I emptied my bowels and cleaned myself. I noted that the toilet paper was bloodstained and discarded it into the toilet. Up to this point I had endured very little pain, other than when I was told to 'let the air out', but the pain I had just experienced was like none before.

I returned to my bed, lying beside my wife. She was clearly shocked and asked me repeatedly whether I was alright. I assured her I was, telling her there was now no pain, thankfully.

So, we both waited, very impatiently. My wife was very reassuring, confirming to me that everything would be fine and she would return later after my surgery. Minutes later, the anaesthetist, Dr Becker, entered the room. He explained to me the procedure he would be undertaking, further explaining that, although my operation was to be performed manually, it was being performed by one of the best surgeons in his chosen field in the country. Again, I felt confident and he relaxed me the best he could before leaving the room.

At approximately 09:00, Mr Syed entered. I told him of my latest enema experience and he stated there would be no need for any further enemas. He told me that during the surgery he would make sure everything was in order in that area. His visit was brief, but my time was now rapidly approaching.

What seemed like an hour passed, but it was, in fact, only around ten minutes before another visitor entered the room. His name was Andy and he was to take me to theatre. My wife and I walked with him along corridors before descending in several lifts. As we walked, Andy pointed out different wards to us. It was like a guided tour of the local hospital, although little of it registered with me as I had other things on my mind. We reached a room which Andy called the 'holding bay,' although he explained that officially he wasn't allowed to call it that. It was a small room outside the operating theatre. I hugged my wife and we said our goodbyes before I was led into theatre.

Mr Syed, Dr Becker and several other people were present, all dressed in surgical gowns, masks and gloves; my resting place for the next hours was situated in the centre of the room.

I was invited to lie on my back on the bed. It was now almost time to say goodbye to my invader. I smiled inwardly, whilst chatting to Dr Becker, although I am unable to recall what was said. My heart was now racing, partly through fear and partly through excitement. The time had come, after the months of fear, anxiety and pain, for my invader to be banished. I would not miss him. In a month or two, I would have recovered. He would be no more and would probably be sitting in a jar of chemicals in some laboratory or incinerated beyond recognition. My invader had caused me so much trauma and now his time was up. I hoped our paths would never cross again.

As I lay, prostrate on the bed, Dr Becker placed a plastic mask over my nose and mouth.

'I'm going to put you to sleep now,' were his last words to me.

I hoped it wasn't going to be permanent! I needn't have worried. I never saw Dr Becker again.

CHAPTER SIX

Much Talking, Much Snoring and Much Morphine

I awoke in a large room containing between twenty and thirty beds which were mostly occupied. My stomach area was covered in various medical dressings and I was attached to several machines including an electrocardiogram (ECG) to monitor my heart rate, which was held in place by the obligatory suction cups attached to my chest. Clipped to the bottom of my nose was a tube to monitor my oxygen level and a catheter was inserted into my urethra, allowing me to urinate into a drainage bag without even realising.

There were several nurses attending to various patients and it was the typical hustle and bustle of any hospital ward you'd expect. There was just one subtle difference: it was extremely quiet, due to the lack of visitors, and the 'clients' were mainly sleeping off their various medications.

I was not in any defining pain. I felt sleepy and lethargic but pain, at this point, was not an issue. What I did suffer from was a severe itchiness in both my legs. This ran all the way from each thigh to each ankle and I guessed it had something to do with the various drugs that had entered my bloodstream in the previous hours. I began scratching my legs vigorously. My scratching obviously alerted a nurse who approached and enquired how I was feeling. I told her I felt OK but had severe itching. She was not phased and checked the levels of the various machines attached to my body, which were displayed on the screen. My feet, by this time, were protruding from the sheets and she remarked on the length of the nail on my right big toe.

'You've got a right nail going on there,' she remarked, jokingly.

I smiled back, not saying a word. In all the preparation prior to my hospital visit I had forgotten to cut my toenails! I was not embarrassed by her observation. By now, I had experienced various objects being inserted up me, down me and into me by various individuals and the nurse was commenting on the length of one of my toenails!

Having checked and recorded what she needed to, the nurse left, clearly amused by my toenail. Thankfully, over a short time, the itchiness in my legs began to fade and I slowly became more alert.

After several hours, two hospital porters arrived and my bed and I were wheeled away from the recovery ward along several corridors and into the surgical high care unit. Immediately I took a dislike to my new home. It was much smaller than the ward I had just left and much busier. Alarms from the various medical machines seemed to be sounding left, right and centre and the place was the opposite of peaceful. Nurses and doctors were hurrying around visiting various patients whose privacy was only protected by a thin piece of material, the curtain which had been pulled around their beds. I could hear almost every word which was being exchanged between nurses and patients, and their privacy was only marginally protected.

I lay there watching the curtains being opened and closed, and nurses entering and exiting. Thankfully, my bed had been pushed into one of the corners of the room, so I only had one neighbour who was to my left-hand side. He was sleeping peacefully and was silent apart from his snoring! He was oblivious to all around him with his curtains closed; each time he breathed in, the decibel levels in the room shot up! He seemed to be taking in so much air I expected the thin curtains surrounding him to be ripped from their fastenings and disappear into his, clearly, wide open mouth! They didn't.

Another patient, approximately three beds to my left, kept talking. He wasn't talking to anyone in particular, just talking. He was visited several times by two nurses who closed the 'privacy' curtains behind them. From their conversations, it became apparent that 'Mr Talk A Lot' was an alcoholic and this wasn't his first visit to this ward. I felt sorry for him. From his words, he was clearly an intelligent man. Fate had conspired against him. Perhaps he'd fallen on difficult times or perhaps he'd recently lost someone dear to him. I didn't know. Although I felt pity for him, it didn't stop me thinking to myself, 'I wish he'd shut the fuck up!' He didn't!

My wife and son visited me during the late afternoon.

Clearly, they were shocked at seeing someone so emotionally close to them lying in a hospital bed with various machines attached to them. I assured them I was doing OK, which was true. I wasn't in any significant pain, just uncomfortable. When it came time for them to leave, they were clearly more reassured than when they arrived.

That night I barely slept. 'Mr Snore A lot' and 'Mr Talk A Lot' saw to that, along with the various alarms being activated seemingly each minute. Various medicines and painkillers were administered to me and the other patients at regular intervals during the night. It seemed that as soon as I managed to pluck a few moments of sleep from the disturbances, I was awoken by some activity or noise taking place. If it wasn't snoring or talking, it was the sound of an alarm from one of the hospital machines.

All I longed for was to leave this ward and be taken to the Nelson Suite where I could enjoy some peace and quiet. That may well sound like an extremely selfish statement, and it is, but that was exactly how I felt. I just wanted my own room where I could lie and sleep when I wished, waking only when necessary.

The following day eventually arrived, after an almost sleepless night. I hadn't eaten or drunk anything since the night before my surgery and didn't relish the idea of doing so. There was a drip attached to the cannula, which had been inserted into the large vein in the top of my right hand which, I assumed, fed me any hydration I needed. Food was the last thing on my mind. I had no appetite for either food or drink.

I just wanted to rest and sleep but, sadly, both were in short supply.

During the morning I received two visitors. The first was a physiotherapist. She explained that I needed to be up on my feet as soon as was physically possible and walking a few paces was extremely important. She, along with a nurse, helped me from my bed. With the physiotherapist supporting me on one side and me holding the mobile drip stand on the other, I managed to walk around five meters from my bed, dragging my drip post with me. My steps were short and deliberate, and I found them difficult. Still, I returned to my bed with a small sense of pride. I had been told I would need six to eight weeks of recuperation following surgery and these small steps were the first on that journey. I was still in no real pain and just had an uncomfortable feeling around my stomach area. I felt proud and elated that I had accomplished today's 'ramble' and, as I lay on my bed, I felt a great sense of joy. My intruder had been forcibly removed as he wouldn't leave of his own accord and he was gone – forever. My life which he had curtailed over the last six months or so could begin again very soon. That was the plan I hatched; however, that wasn't to be. We all know life has a way of throwing you a curveball!

A short while later, a nurse approached, wheeling a small table. A cup of something warm was upon it.

'I'd like you to try and drink this,' she remarked.

I sat up, the nurse offering me a helping hand, and I could

see the contents within the cup. It was half full of black tea, no sugar, no milk. On the tabletop next to the cup was a cardboard sick bowl.

I managed to sip from the cup several times. I took maybe three or four tablespoon-size amounts but, within a second of my last sip, the sick bowl was in use! It seemed that at least four or five times the amount I consumed left my mouth, much more rapidly than it had entered, sitting gently in the bottom of the cardboard vessel.

The nurse then explained how important it was for me to drink although, now laying my head back on my pillow, I wasn't really listening. I was then offered more of the black liquid which, funnily enough, I declined.

My next visit was during the morning. A doctor came to my bed, carrying a clipboard. He thumbed through the notes, asking me various questions, to which I answered as best I could. Once he finished his questioning, I questioned him.

'When can I go to the Nelson Suite, Doctor?' I asked.

He looked straight into my eyes and his reply was blunt.

'You are receiving the best care in this ward this hospital has to offer,' he replied.

With this said he seemed to spin quickly around on the balls of his feet and walked rapidly away, holding the clipboard tightly in his right hand. As he left the room, I imagined him muttering derogatory words to himself about private patients. Clearly my question upset him.

I immediately realised my question was a selfish one. I wished I could close my privacy curtains around my bed, pull the sheets over my head and disappear for a while but I couldn't, so I just lay sheepishly where I was, regretting my questioning of the doctor. I didn't mean to upset him in any way. I just wished for some peace so I could attempt to rest without listening to the dulcet tones of 'Mr Talk A Lot' and 'Mr Snore A Lot'.

Later that afternoon, my wish was granted. Like a genie released from the bottle, a nurse approached.

'We're going to move you shortly, Mr Michaels', she explained 'To the Nelson Suite.'

Within minutes, two hospital porters arrived and I was being wheeled away, out of the ward, into a large elevator which took us to the top floor of the hospital. I was pushed along a short corridor towards a double door with a sign displayed above it, reading: Welcome to the Nelson Suite.

The doors were keypad entry only, automatically locking as they closed behind us. I was wheeled past the room where I had experienced my fateful enema. We turned left, passed the nurses' station and then turned right, into a room which was to be my 'home' for the foreseeable future.

The room was sparsely furnished. It had a small armchair adjacent to the window, a tall, but thin, bedside cabinet containing several drawers which was pushed against the wall. There was a chair, which resembled a dining room chair, next to a small, mobile, tray table on which was a white electric fan. There was a compact television on an extendable bracket fixed to the wall, and programmes could be purchased if so desired.

My bed was wheeled into position along with my mobile drip post. Both were positioned against the wall between the television and the cabinet. I noticed that directly opposite the bed was a bathroom which housed a small walk-in shower and a single basin with taps. A white porcelain toilet was set against the wall facing the bathroom door.

So there I lay, cannula in the vein on top of my right hand, drip post next to the bed and a catheter inserted into my penis.

As I lay, prostrate on my back, I was overwhelmed by something quite simple. The quietness! I had been moved from a general hospital ward where all the experiences you would expect were taking place. The nurses going about their duties, visitors visiting, doctors appearing before quickly disappearing from bedsides, medical machines alarms seemingly being activated by the minute, 'Mr Talk A Lot' and 'Mr Snore A Lot' continuing to expel their sounds and the sound of curtains being pulled around bedsides before being pulled open once more.

There was none of that. Very little noise at all. Every now and then a figure would pass by the open door to my room, before returning in the opposite direction. There was not the hustle and bustle as there had been in the surgical high care unit.

I lay, completely alone, drip attached, staring out of the large window which overlooked the city. It was now 8th May

2016 and the early summer sunshine lit up the houses and businesses below. No hustle and no bustle, just peace and quiet but, peculiarly, a little piece of me missed the busyness of the previous ward I had spent time in.

I dozed on and off most of the afternoon, only waking to the visiting nurses checking on my condition and feeding me the various pills and liquids I was required to take at these times.

A further visit from the physiotherapist and another short walk followed. A visit from my wife, then more dozing, and my second day in hospital was drawing to a close.

Upon a further visit from a nurse, I was informed that my temperature was somewhat high and a portable air conditioning unit was supplied to cool me down. It seemed to work and any anxieties felt by the nurses or myself quickly diminished.

Around 22:00, a nurse entered my room. She was of Filipino appearance and she held the last tablet of the day for me in her hand. It was a single, small white tablet which I swallowed without question. Well, I can tell you, it was the best tablet I have ever taken! Within minutes, I felt like I was floating. It took any pain or discomfort rapidly from my body and I could feel myself smiling broadly, almost laughing out loud, before I fell into a deep sleep.

Apparently, during the early hours, I used my mobile telephone and rang my wife. I was speaking nonsense to her and to this day I don't recall the conversation or even making the call. Clearly the side-effects of my last pill of the day, my lovely morphine tablet, were very noticeable!

The next morning, I awoke early from my slumber and waited for the first visit of the day. I didn't have to wait long before the door to my room was opened and in came the nurse. She gave me several tablets, which I consumed, before giving me another beautiful morphine tablet and I fell back to sleep, smiling once more!

Two days after my operation, the oxygen monitor and ECG monitor were removed, along with my drip and the mobile drip stand. My strength began to return and I was able to leave my bed of my own accord and venture, slowly, out of my room to undertake my twice-daily short walks along the corridor and back again.

I received visits from friends and family, and each day I felt stronger. There were no further dramas and three days after my surgery, my catheter was removed. I had heard stories that when this procedure takes place it can be a very painful affair, so I was anxious when the nurse entered my room and informed me she was going to remove it.

I needn't have worried. It took seconds to remove. I barely felt any discomfort, let alone any pain. Again, the *thought* of having something done to me far outweighed the actual action.

I was now eating and drinking well, polishing off full meals, although a restriction was put on the amount of fruit and vegetables I was allowed to consume. Gone were the first few days of only eating small amounts of soup and water. My appetite had now returned and, along with it, my strength.

I would sit in the armchair by the window, just staring out, watching the world pass, the May sunshine warming the room as it passed through the glass. The minutes passed by, turning into hours. I visited the toilet when needed, although I was still unable to open my bowels.

Now I was gaining in strength, seemingly hourly, taking my slow, deliberate walks, visiting the bathroom to wash and urinate. I was feeling confident that my hospital stay was drawing to a close. The amount of medication I was taking was declining and the 'magic' morphine pills had, unfortunately, ceased. Everything in my world now felt good. Visits from loved ones cheered me, no end. These included my wife, mother and father, John, my wife's father, and my brother-in-law Matthew, along with my good friend and work colleague, Patrick.

Wednesday 11th May 2016 arrived. I was sitting by the window watching the busy world pass by, when, from the corner of my eye, I saw a figure enter the room. I turned my head as the figure came closer. I recognised him immediately. It was the surgeon who had removed my invader, ultimately saving my life, 'Smoky Eyes,' Mr Syed. I was so pleased to see him and shook his hand vigorously, thanking him from the bottom of my heart for what he'd done. The thanks I gave him were not just words. I meant them emphatically, after all, it was due to his huge skill in his chosen field that I was living and breathing. He had removed the demon from within me, allowing my life to continue and to enjoy life, enabling me to hug my loved ones and joke with my friends. I knew I would always be eternally grateful to him and his team for what they had done.

Pleasantries followed and we jovially spoke about cricket before thoughts turned to my surgery. He explained that all had gone well during the procedure and that he had made five small incisions around my navel. There was one to the left of my navel, one to the right, three above it and one actually into it. The main incision was then made between my navel and my pubic line, just below where I would fasten my trousers. This main incision was horizontal, around four to five inches long and about a quarter of an inch thick. He explained that the scarring from the main incision would probably always be visible. However, the scarring from the smaller incisions would almost certainly disappear completely in time. I had seen the smaller incisions whilst my dressing was being changed, but I was yet to see the larger one due to its position. Any scarring was the absolute least of my worries and a very small price to pay for the removal of my tumour which had caused such pain and anguish to me and my loved ones.

Mr Syed continued, explaining that the procedure had lasted around three-and-a-half to four hours, and that he had removed the contaminated part of my lower bowel. He demonstrated the length of the part he had removed by holding his arms out in front of him and parting his hands. I was shocked by how far his hands were parted. It appeared that he had removed around eight to ten inches of my lower bowel. The two un-joined ends were then forcibly stapled back together and, due to the stapling, my lower bowel would be stronger than prior to the procedure. Having removed the infected part of my lower bowel, he explained that I did not need a stoma (colostomy bag) for temporary or permanent use. Once I was discharged from hospital, I would need around four to six weeks to recover. He stated that I would be discharged once I had opened my bowels and confirmed that I could eat what I desired, although not too much fruit and vegetables for a few weeks. He further explained that, during the surgery, a number of lymph glands had been removed along with part of my lower bowel. These glands acted as filters through which the blood flowed and these would be analysed. Once he received the results of this analysis, he would contact me.

We said our farewells and I shook his hand once more, thanked him again, before watching him leave the room. I then stumbled my way slowly to the toilet in the vain hope of passing just a very small lump of excretion. Despite vigorous efforts, nothing budged! How ironic, I thought. For the previous five or six months, I had willed that nothing would leave my body via my rear and now I was struggling to even make the smallest amount exit my body!

That evening, I managed to shower, avoiding as best I could the warm water splashing onto the dressing that covered my wounds. After showering, I went for my short walk along the corridor, managing to cover around thirty metres or so. After chatting to several nurses at the nurses' station, I began my return journey. My steps were very slow and ponderous – I was travelling at the speed you'd expect someone twice my age to travel at. Progress was progress and it was what it was.

I was still swallowing several pills a day along with medicine which was injected directly into my stomach area. However, I knew my discharge would be soon and I would be able to enjoy my home comforts once more.

My life over the past five months or so had been a series of peaks and troughs, mainly troughs! For the first time since my problems began, I felt myself leaving the bottom of the trough and quickly heading towards the peak. Cancer had blighted my life for what seemed an age but now that cancer was gone and I was looking forward to continuing my life once again, picking it back up from where I had left it all those months previously.

That evening my cannula was removed, just leaving the top of my right hand bruised and slightly sore. It was the last piece of medical 'machinery' which had been attached to me to be removed. I was not unhappy to see the large needle pulled from my vein before being swiftly discarded into a nearby 'sharps' bin.

I slept well that night in the hope that the next day I would open my bowels, leading to two discharges, the second being from the hospital!

The next morning, I was awoken by the delivery of my small breakfast, followed by a visit from the nurse. I was given some tablets, received an injection and took a quick shower. Two toilet visits followed, without any success, and a short hobble to the nurses' station followed. I returned and slowly lowered myself into the armchair by the window in my room.

Another unsuccessful toilet visit followed, then lunch, before a further visit to the toilet. I had now decided to remain positioned until something, no matter how small, stirred within me. Eventually it did! Following much pushing and panting, the success I had longed for occurred. A lump the size of a marble left me, broke the surface of the still water and sank in the blink of an eye. I felt like I had passed something the size of a tennis ball, but I hadn't. My 'marble' was more akin to a garden pea than a tennis ball and remained in situ, almost staring back at me. I smiled, wiped, stood and flushed 'him' away. It had been the first time in a long time that only faeces had left my body and thanks to my 'marble,' my peak was now much nearer.

I reported the results immediately to the nurse who was sat at her station. She was clearly pleased for me, raising both thumbs and offering me a broad smile. I returned to my room, positioned myself in the armchair where I had spent so much time over the past few days, and continued to watch a small part of the world go by.

A short while later, a nurse entered, wanting to change my dressing. I assumed the position, prostrate on the bed. My dressing had been changed no end of times during my stay but this time something was different. The nurse was spending more time than usual examining my main wound.

By the look on her face, she appeared concerned.

'What the hell now,' I thought to myself, before the nurse provided an answer.

'I am afraid it appears your wound is infected, Mr Michaels.'

My heart immediately sank. I was unable to respond as she continued.

'Don't worry, we'll make sure everything will be OK.'

The nurse explained that I had a small amount of liquid literally dripping from my larger wound. It was something I had been unable to see as I lay prone and she continued cleaning and dressing the area. Within a minute or two, my dressings were complete and she left the room briefly, before returning once more. My heart was now racing. What the hell did this mean? Would I need to stay in hospital longer? Would I be facing further medical procedures due to my infection? Was it serious? My ignorance was breeding my fear once more.

It was explained to me that these types of infections were actually more common than people anticipated. I was still to be discharged later that day and was to be supplied with syringes, pain killers and anti-sickness medicine. The injections were to be self-administered for three weeks and I would need to finish the course of the other medicines I would be given. I would need to make an appointment to see the nurse at my local health centre the following day. There, the nurse would clean my wound and change my dressings. I would be prescribed antibiotics which, it was hoped, would cure my infection.

Thanks to the nurse's words, I was not now unduly worried about my infection. After all, over the past weeks and months I had fought a much stronger, more powerful enemy and had been victorious. No infection was going to change that result. I would take the medicines, visit the nurse at the health centre, rest and recuperate for the following weeks and months. Although I would have a scar to show for the rest of my life, that would be it. I was free from the enemy within, the enemy which had blighted my life for what seemed so long now. I was looking forward to my life continuing, being able to enjoy experiences once more and maybe find some new ventures.

As I sat in my armchair, watching the world pass by, I became overjoyed by the thought that in the very near future the handbrake that had been applied all those months previously was soon to be released.

During the late afternoon, my wife arrived and we both waited for my official release. Seconds ticked by, turning into minutes then hours. I had dressed myself earlier and was just waiting for the nurse to visit and give me my marching orders. A short while later, she did. At 20:00 I was discharged. I said my goodbyes, thanked those who had looked after me so well and, having declined the use of a wheelchair, I left my room, walking slowly along the corridor, passing the nurses' station, through the security doors and out of the Nelson Suite into the main part of the hospital. I immediately felt the hustle and bustle of the main hospital once more. All manner of people were rushing around, beds were being pushed into lifts and nurses were hurrying about their daily business. Other staff members, with their identity tags hanging from their necks, rushed around, here, there and everywhere.

My tranquil life of the past five days was gone, almost instantly. I walked slowly and deliberately away from the private ward into a lift which carried me and my wife to the ground floor. By the time we exited the lift, I was already regretting my decision declining the use of a wheelchair. My pride had forced me into hobbling along at an embarrassingly slow speed. With every step I longed to be seated comfortably whilst being pushed along the meandering corridors.

The journey on foot continued. It was only one of a few hundred metres but it took at least fifteen minutes before I was seated in the passenger seat of my wife's car, taking the short journey back to our home, the small white paper bag of medicines resting in my lap.

The date was 12th May 2016, five days since my operation and five days since being at the mercy of my invader. Life was beginning to feel good once more.

CHAPTER SEVEN

The Call That Changed It All

The following morning arrived after a decent sleep and I made the appointment to see the nurse at my local health centre. The appointment was made for the afternoon and I liaised with my insurers, who were happy for me to seek assistance from the National Health Service.

During the morning I felt liquid of some description oozing from my main wound. The dressing covering my wounds began to feel damp on the inside and the appointment couldn't come soon enough.

My wife and I left in good time as I knew the short walk from the car park to the centre would take at least three or four times longer than normal, due to the fact I was only able to walk at a very slow pace, thanks to my wounds. We arrived at the surgery in good time and I was seen almost immediately. The nurse changed my dressing and I was prescribed the suitable antibiotics, which were to be taken in conjunction with my other medicines. I was supplied with various bandages and dressings and shown how to apply them, in the event that the leakage proved too much for the dressing already in place.

I, naturally, questioned the nurse regarding my infection.

Seeing my obvious concerns, she reassured me. She explained that these types of infections were not uncommon and after a few days my wound would begin to settle and the healing would continue naturally. A further appointment was made for 16th May, three days later.

Naturally, I was concerned that my infection would worsen and cause me further problems. I had never experienced what I had been through before and my ignorance increased the fear within me. Despite these fears, the medical staff I had met and who had treated me so far allayed those fears.

That evening, the dressing needed changing once more. A clear liquid was seeping from the bottom edge of the dressing, dampening the top of the baggy tracksuit bottoms I was wearing. My wife and I made our way upstairs to our bedroom to 'don' the new dressing. Although it had now been seven full days since my surgery, I had not seen my main wound with my own eyes. The only way I could see it was by using a full-length mirror, something which I did not have access to in the hospital.

As my wife started to release the dressing, I was overcome with fear. I dreaded what I was about to see. Again, I was venturing into the unknown and when that happens, a certain amount of fear enters your mind. The unknown is often feared until it is faced. Once faced, the unknown becomes the known and the fear can, only then, begin to diminish.

I had visions of a gaping, open wound, oozing puss and

being abnormally coloured. I felt I would be able to put my finger within it and feel my insides if I so desired. As with so many of the previous experiences of the last months, I needn't have worried.

The dressing was released and there it was, my main wound. It was around four inches long and a quarter of an inch wide, running horizontally, between my naval and pubic line. It appeared to be a light grey in colour. It was completely sealed and looked like someone had taken a thick felt tip pen and drawn a horizontal, straight line, some three inches or so below my navel. Tiny parts of it glistened but there was no flow of liquid and no open, gaping wound. The only thing that really struck me was that along its length the area was indented slightly, as though being pulled from within me. Due to this indent I was unable to see it whilst lying on my back so the only way of viewing it was via a mirror.

The other smaller wounds were visible to me without the use of any aids. They appeared to be healing well, were already scabbed and were much smaller in length, each one being barely half an inch long. They ran in an upward curve from one side of my navel until they reached their peak approximately two inches directly above my navel, before curving down again. Together with my main wound it was as though someone had drawn a semi-circle, the edges of which were broken, on my stomach.

Having seen the 'bottom' of my semi-circle, I was extremely relieved. The ignorance that had bred the fear was becoming all too common on this journey.

There were no further dramas over the weekend. I injected my stomach daily and took my tablets as instructed. The only real problem I was having was opening my bowels. I'd sit on the toilet for a good fifteen to twenty minutes before anything would appear and, when it did, its size was very disappointing! I was taking self-prescribed laxatives but was still struggling until, three days after being discharged from hospital, the floodgates opened. The laxatives had taken their effect, much to the relief of both me and my now much shorter lower bowel.

A visit to the nurse on 16th May led to a new dressing and I continued with the medication, injections and plenty of rest, as I had been instructed. By 20th May, my course of antibiotics had finished and, although my midriff was still leaky, the leaking was much less, clearly slowing gradually. I would find that one day it would weep very slightly and the next it wouldn't leak at all, until finally it completely stopped leaking. The problem was solved! It had now been thirteen days since I underwent surgery.

With the passing of each day, I became stronger and was not suffering pain, just discomfort in my stomach area, which was also becoming less. I still wasn't very mobile, with walking speeds severely reduced but I was now on my feet regularly. I would do a little housework, then rest, then continue. The ups and downs of the last six months were now mainly ups. I was off work and received no pressure to return, which I was very grateful for. I was in regular contact with my good friend, Patrick, and my brother-in-law, Matthew, along with my boss at work. I just rested as and when needed and I felt that, slowly, my life was returning to some sort of normality.

During this time, I received a telephone call, completely unexpectedly, from Dr Richardson, the doctor I had visited first back in April. During our conversation, she was apologetic to me, telling me that she was sorry to hear that I had suffered from bowel cancer. I reassured her that I was now fine and resting after my surgery. I told her that following our meeting I had gone private, only because that option was open to me. In my mind she had done everything correctly, being professional and approachable.

I was quite taken aback that she had taken the time out of very busy schedule to phone me personally. This was something I had never experienced before, and I had total respect for her and the way she had questioned and examined me during our meeting. I also respected her for her telephone call to me. After all, it wasn't her fault that I had developed bowel cancer and she had been completely professional. Upon saying our goodbyes, I said, 'Not seen you in the supermarket yet.'

She giggled, said goodbye and our phone call ended.

My emotional rollercoaster of the last six months now appeared to be rapidly slowing. I had been through my problems and all the emotions they had brought with them: the not knowing what was happening to my body, the fear that ignorance had produced in my mind and the fear which cancer had bestowed on me and my loved ones. It had been a long six months and my body had undergone procedures which I had never even considered, let alone endured. My insides had clearly taken a real beating but what I had undergone had taken me from someone who had been extremely ill with a life-threatening condition to someone who was almost back to full fitness. I realised that I would never be completely 'normal' ever again as my body was now partially incomplete. Part of it had been cut away, along with the 'demon' which is cancer and that missing piece could never be replaced. It was gone and so was the tumour which had blighted my recent life. The cancer had caused emotion and pain not only to me, but to those closest to me. It wasn't just me who had suffered as the cancer had grown slowly but unmistakeably within me. The cancer was like an octopus with 'His' arms reaching out, pulling individuals towards 'Him' without mercy. 'He' was now gone and I was recovering well, getting stronger each day, slowly returning to the normality I had longed for over such a long period now.

I was grateful that I would soon be living my life properly once more. Those closest to me had been loving and supportive throughout this sad chapter of my life. They also suffered but I will never know how much. My 'demon' within had laid out 'His' battle plans against me but with the medical professionals as my generals, the 'demon' had lost.

Of course, I realised that I had become one of the lucky ones who had been touched by cancer, but not overwhelmed by it. In my mind, Mr C had visited and had begun to weave 'His' particular kind of 'magic' but, for some reason, ceased his weaving before finishing 'His' work. Why was that? With so many 'He' completes 'His' task but, with me, 'He' had visited only briefly as though just passing through, saying a brief hello before visiting some other poor soul to torment. I had already learnt so much from 'Him'. Things I had never even thought of, experiences I could only have imagined. One thing I learnt was that being diagnosed with cancer wasn't a death sentence. It was a battle, yes, but it was winnable. Many had lost their battles and many had won.

Who knows why 'He' hadn't stayed – I don't, but I was glad 'He' had gone. Or had 'He'?

The days passed without incident and it was now over two weeks since my surgery. It was a very special day in the Michaels' household. It was 22nd May 2016 and both my son's and daughter's birthdays. Both were born on the same day, four years apart. It was my daughter's twenty-first and my son's seventeenth. I recalled their births well. My daughter was born quickly, within three hours of the onset of labour. However, it was a different story regarding my son. He was overdue and a number of false alarms had occurred prior to his appearance. He waited until the clock ticked midnight and the 21st became the 22nd. Three minutes later he was here, brought into the world by my loving wife and a loving midwife. It was as though he knew it was his older sister's birthday and he offered her the most important of presents: a sibling.

So, both birthdays on the same day and always a special time for the parents. We had a small gathering at our house with close family. Presents were exchanged and love and laughter ran throughout our small, detached home. A cake was presented to each of my children and they both blew out a single candle which had been inserted into the centre. It was a happy day for all of us.

I was grateful I was able to enjoy their day and glad that the peaks and troughs of the last half year had now, mainly, become peaks. My infection had been resolved and I had finished taking my tablet medication, although I was still injecting my stomach and would do so for about a further week. Life had become good. I was not working whilst undergoing my recuperation and the pressure of work was not upon me. The brakes on my emotional roller coaster were now rigidly applied and I felt I was almost at the summit of my own personal Mount Everest. The journey had begun, just as any journey does with those initial small steps which had now grown in size. Although physically unable, mentally I was running towards the mountain top. I felt nothing could now stop me from summiting that mountain. Its summit had been so high, so out of reach, covered in clouds and invisible to me when my journey had begun. Now it was truly visible, within my grasp. My journey of uncertainty, anguish and fear was coming to an end. The light at the end of the tunnel began shining brightly and I was running quicker and quicker towards the light of normality, closely followed by my loved ones who had also been affected by my illness. We could all enter the light together, summit the mountain together and rejoice as one.

The following day began as normal but would prove to be

anything but a normal day. Breakfast was consumed, followed by my daily injection. My wife left for work around 08:30, just as she did each working day. I did a little housework, then assumed my prone position on the couch, enjoying my well-earned rest, falling into a light sleep with the sun shining through the window onto my body, warming me and helping with the snoozing process.

I was awoken by the telephone's high-pitched ringing tone breaking the solace. I moved slowly from my position to answer the call.

'Hello, Anthony Michaels,' I said, somewhat formally as I noticed the incoming call was from a withheld number. There was a short pause before a voice I knew well and immediately recognised sounded in my ear.

'Good morning, Anthony,' Mr Syed replied.

Formalities over, 'Smoky Eyes' enquired about my health and how I was feeling. I assured him I was doing well, taking my medication as prescribed and resting as I should. He was as professional and reassuring as always and, as we spoke, I began to sense there was a more important reason for his call. I was right.

'Do you remember that I told you that during your surgery I removed and examined a number of glands which were attached to the part of your bowel I removed?' he asked.

My reply was short.

'Yes I do.' I was now becoming nervous.

'Well,' he continued, 'those lymph nodes act as filters for the blood. I removed twenty-four of them from the infected area and one of them showed signs of cancer.'

By now I knew what he was about to tell me.

'Unfortunately, you will need to undergo a course of chemotherapy which I will discuss with one of the oncologists here and he will contact you shortly to arrange an appointment. However, I will see you prior to that to check on your progress.'

With that, we wished each other well and the call ended.

I assumed my resting position once more. However, sleep was now the last thing on my mind. CHEMOTHERAPY! The very word scared me – I had very little knowledge about it and my ignorance, again, bred a multitude of fears within me. I had never experienced chemotherapy, only hearing about it second-hand during conversations and seeing images of people who had undergone treatment. Those images alone were enough to make me frightened, let alone having to undergo the treatment myself.

Images of women, looking pale and gaunt, with little or no hair, filled my mind. For some reason, which I am unable to explain, it was only images of women that filled my mind. Pale women, thin women, women wearing bandanas and looking very ill and very weak, filled my thoughts. I could not think of any images of men that had had or were undergoing chemotherapy. Perhaps I had never even seen any males of the human race receiving this kind of treatment. I racked my brain, but the only pictures I could raise were of those 'poor' women who always, always looked so ill, with tubes entering their bodies, carrying the chemicals that produced those heart-breaking images. These pictures were etched into my mind. Didn't males undergo such treatment? Of course they did, but still no images of them came to mind.

So, what choice did I have now? It was simple. I could undergo the dreaded chemotherapy or refuse it. If I underwent treatment, there was a good chance I would make a complete recovery but if I refused, I could possibly die a very painful death. The latter didn't really enter my mind. Again, it was what it was. Mr C had visited and trashed part of my insides before being evicted, but 'His' ghost, 'His' spirit, had remained. 'His' presence was still with me and a small strand of His' web was still being weaved and still inflicting its damage.

I had undergone my 'problems,' experienced lifesaving surgery, become infected, weak and drained, and then I had begun my recovery. Now, 'He' had returned wearing a large pair of steel toe-capped boots and kicked me swiftly between the legs! That was how I felt. All the ups and downs of the past six months had come and gone but the brakes on my emotional rollercoaster had now been fully disengaged and a brand-new journey was beginning. The chemotherapy journey had been given the green light and, again, the fearful unknown was upon me. Ignorance was once more breeding fear.

I waited until my wife returned from work before I broke the news to her and we held each other tightly. Again, she reassured and supported me. She, once again, had to endure more bad news thanks to my 'visitor' and my heart went out to her. She was strong and always had been. However, I worried about how my news would impact upon her and the rest of my loved ones.

My journey was my journey, but I knew that those travelling with me would also be affected. The journey had to be continued until the destination was reached and we would all feel the bumps and potholes in the road. No matter how large the bumps, or how deep the holes, I knew that journey would have to continue.

Over the following days, I liaised with my insurers and learnt that the cost of any private treatment was covered by them so I wouldn't have to worry about any of the expense. The only items not covered were things like painkillers. Anti-sickness medicines, steroid treatment, chemotherapy and radiotherapy expenses would be paid for by them. The insurers also had a telephone line to a team of trained cancer nurses, whom I could call on if needed for reassurance, guidance or just generally talk to should I feel the need, which offered some comfort to me.

On 2nd June2016, I had a further appointment with 'Smoky Eyes' at the private hospital. By now I had finished my medication and my 'wounds' were uncovered. He was happy with my progress and gave me some insight into what to expect from chemotherapy. He explained that my cancer was now classed as Stage 3. For those who are unaware:

Stage 1 cancer means the cancer is small and confined to

one area.

Stage 2 cancer means the cancer has grown and is growing but hasn't affected other areas or organs.

Stage 3 cancer means the cancer has grown further, with a wider spread, and cancer cells may have been detected in the lymph nodes.

Stage 4 cancer means the cancer has spread from where it originated into another organ. This is also known as metastatic or secondary cancer.

As cancer cells had been detected within one of the twenty-four lymph nodes removed, my cancer was now classed as Stage 3. Mr Syed explained that chemotherapy was needed to destroy any existing cancer cells which may have travelled through my lymph nodes into my blood stream and possibly into any organs. He concluded by advising me that I may suffer from some side-effects, but the oncologist would be able to explain in greater detail the treatment involved and any side-effects from that treatment.

The following day I received a call from a lady called Julie, who was the secretary to Dr Patel, the oncologist who would be treating me. An appointment was made for me to meet him at the private hospital on 7th June 2016, at 19:00. It was a meeting that, peculiarly, I was looking forward to. I would be able to learn more from that one short meeting about my future treatment than I had learnt from my (almost) 50 years of life. I hoped, with a little knowledge, my fear would not run so deep. I was completely ignorant of chemotherapy which expanded my fear incredibly. Ignorance, once again, had bread fear.

On this same day, I also had a visitor to my home. My boss arrived for a coffee and a 'catch up.' He brought with him an official-looking letter which explained that he would continue to pay me my salary over the following weeks and months. I was to be paid in full whether I was at work or not. It was an offer I gladly accepted and eased my financial worries. Obviously, I didn't want to have the worry about money whilst I was off work. It was something that had occurred to me briefly but was not at the forefront of my mind as I had my health to worry about. It meant that, until I returned to work, which I knew would be on a part-time basis initially, financially I would have some security, for which I was very grateful.

The day of my meeting with the oncologist arrived. In the early evening, my wife drove us to the hospital for my rendezvous with Dr Patel. Again we positioned ourselves in the waiting room, watching the clock on the wall slowly tick. It seemed that whenever I was seated in this room, time seemed to slow and the longer I sat, the slower the ticking became!

Seven o'clock, the time of my appointment, came and went. I thought to myself, 'Here we go again, more waiting.' I knew I was being impatient and selfish and I reminded myself of the reasons I had been kept waiting on my first visit to see 'Smoky Eyes.' With these thoughts, my patience returned. Ironically, my patience having been restored, a smartly dressed gentleman of Indian appearance, aged in his early forties, with jet black short hair, ventured from one of the corridors and called my name.

My wife and I rose as one, following Dr Patel to a small office along the right-hand corridor. We entered and found ourselves seated on the opposite side of a small desk from the doctor. He introduced himself and I immediately felt at ease in his presence, although I had many fears in the forefront of my mind.

He enquired about my health, to which I replied that my recovery from surgery seemed to be going well, although I was still nowhere near as mobile as I was prior to my operation. He confirmed that I needed to rest as much as possible. He then began telling me the reasons for my upcoming chemotherapy. I learnt that my treatment would last six months and I would have a chemotherapy cycle every two weeks. He explained that following each treatment, I may feel ill for around five days but should then recover from any feelings of nausea. The chemicals were to be administered into my body via something called a peripherally inserted central catheter, known as a PICC line. This is a very thin tube which would be inserted into a vein on the inside of my arm at the elbow, just below my bicep muscle. The tube would then be pushed along the vein, towards my shoulder, across the top of my chest, eventually stopping very near to my heart. The PICC line would then remain in situ for the duration of my treatment. He further explained that, because the line ended near my heart, it meant that any medicines administered intravenously would be pumped rapidly and efficiently into my bloodstream and around my body.

Following each chemotherapy session at the hospital, a pump would be fitted to the PICC line at its entry and further chemicals would continue to be pumped into my body, until its contents were emptied into my system. This pump would be removed when empty, some forty-six hours later. A return to the hospital would then be needed to remove the pump.

The treatment I would undergo was called FOLFOX. This was the treatment for colorectal cancer and included folinic acid, fluorouracil and oxaliplatin. All new words to me!

Dr Patel pointed out that I may suffer several side-effects following the treatment which included sickness, diarrhoea, fatigue and sores growing inside my mouth. Tremendous, I thought to myself. I knew I could suffer side-effects but what he told me next had never entered my mind.

Whilst undergoing treatment, he told me that I should not take anything from the fridge or freezer without either wearing gloves or covering my fingers with some sort of protection. He explained that the nerves in my fingers would be adversely affected and handling anything cold without protection could cause me great pain. This was getting worse by the second.

It was further explained that a number of other side-effects were possible. These ranged from severe hiccups to severe pain in my jaw when chewing. He then stated that these were the most common side-effects and that I may suffer from all of them, some of them, or none of them at all.

I was puzzled and trying to process all the information he was supplying me with. Would I suffer greatly or not at all? I questioned him about this. He replied that we, as humans, were all different and we all reacted differently to treatment, some suffering worse than others and some, although very few, actually suffered from no side-effects whatsoever.

This was all amazing to me. Again, prior to my appointment with Dr Patel, I realised how little I knew, but in this short meeting I had learnt so much.

Following the doctor's outpouring of information, to which I had mainly remained silent trying to comprehend what he was telling me, he asked if I had any questions. Prior to our meeting, I had plenty of questions, but now, with all the information floating around my mind, these questions were gone. I asked him the only question I could think of.

'Will my hair fall out?' I asked him quizzically. Even before I had finished the question, I felt stupid. Just imagine, I was told all about the terrible experiences my body would undergo having been pumped full of chemicals and the only thing I seemed worried about was my hair! Oh, how vain he must have thought I was!

The corners of the doctor's mouth turned slightly up.

'Your hair shouldn't fall out,' he replied. He had obviously been asked this question countless times. 'If you do lose any hair,' he continued, 'which is very unlikely, I can assure you it will grow back, probably even thicker and stronger than it was, although possibly different in colour.'

'Was he now taking the piss?' I thought.

'Don't worry, Mr Michaels' he said, clearly seeing the nervousness in my face. He carried on, pointing out that he was there to treat me, to prescribe the medicines which would be administered by the nurses, and that my quality of life during this treatment was also a priority. Yes, I needed treating, yes, it would take at least twelve cycles over at least six months, and yes, I may suffer some harrowing side-effects, but he was also there to make sure those side-effects would be kept under control, kept as minimal as was possible by the use of numerous other medicines such as anti-sickness medicines and steroids.

Unfortunately, he hadn't convinced me fully and I left the hospital already fearing what my body was soon to undergo. This was all new to me, as it would be to anyone undertaking this kind of treatment for the first time. Although I left the hospital fearful of the next six months or so, due to my ignorance, there was a question that still did not for one millisecond, enter my mind – namely, would I die? There was no way I would even entertain this thought. Again, it was what it was. I needed the treatment and, although fearful of it, I would undergo it. In my mind I had no choice, so I reconciled myself to the fact that my journey was continuing. The road on this journey was going to be a bumpy one with various potholes along the way but it was a journey which I knew would end one day. Unfortunately, that day now seemed a long way away.

CHAPTER EIGHT

The Insertion

So, once more, cancer had dealt not only 'His' subject a devastating blow, but those closest to that subject were also to suffer. Once again, I had to tell my elderly, frail parents terrible news. Their youngest son was due to undergo chemotherapy, having recently undergone lifesaving surgery. My wife and children had to endure the consequences of Mr C once more. Although thankfully 'He' had not seen fit to visit them personally, they still suffered 'His' torment through no fault of their own. Friends and colleagues were told my news and they too were forced by 'Him' to worry for me. Cancer had again weaved a huge web, capturing friends and loved ones, holding them in limbo, forcing their suffering and not allowing them to escape 'His' clutches.

It was as though my unwelcome visitor had entered my world and cast the first blow. I had retaliated with a flurry of blows, enough to make 'Him' take a step back when, without warning, 'He' had produced a further weapon, one invisible to me, inflicting further anguish and pain and forcing me to retreat. My weapon against 'Him' was now poison, in the form of my upcoming treatment. To push 'Him' back to the point of defeat would cause pain and anguish to myself and my loved ones. I was the driver heading towards my destination but my passengers were close by.

Two days later I had a blood test at the private hospital. I then received an appointment to see Dr Patel on 14th June 2016. The day before this appointment, I received a telephone call from a lady called Katherine. She was the nurse in charge of the oncology ward where I was to undergo my treatment. I could tell immediately, just from the way she spoke, that she was extremely caring. Sometimes it is clear in the words which are said, and the way they are said, that they come from the heart.

She confirmed that my PICC line was to be inserted on the 20th June and the following day my dreaded six months of treatment would begin. I say dreaded because I was dreading it. I had not dreaded my previous surgery as it had removed something physical which had been causing problems that were obvious and visible. Once my surgery was completed, I believed that would be the end of my invader. I could recover and continue with my life. Chemotherapy most definitely was not in those plans. My cancer was now invisible to me and wasn't causing me any obvious problems. It was as though chemotherapy was to become part of my recovery, not to remove something physical, but as a second line of defence. Of course, I needed treatment and I accepted that but I was frightened of that treatment and the effect it would have on my body and mind. Again and again, my ignorance increased my fears. The fear of undergoing something sometimes outweighs its actual undergoing, an experience that was becoming all too familiar to me.

A few days after my telephone conversation, my confidence got the better of me. I decided I would drive the short distance to see my granddaughter and daughter. They lived approximately six miles from me. I had been advised to only drive very short distances by medical staff whilst recovering from surgery, due to the position the body is in whilst driving. I had taken their advice and was still taking it as I set off on my short journey. Of course, I had seen both my daughter and granddaughter on several occasions since my operation so I felt sure the journey would not be problematic. I waited until rush hour had passed before setting off. No problems; the journey took the normal time, around fifteen minutes, and support and love continued to flow from my daughter during my visit. Before long, I was heading back home to the comfort of my couch.

Whilst travelling along a short section of dual carriageway, not too far from home, the traffic ground to an abrupt halt. There I sat, as a minute ticked by, then another. Sirens filled the air, seemingly from all directions. It soon became clear that there had been a traffic collision ahead. 'Twos and blues' were heard and seen frantically cutting their way through the traffic to the site of the collision. I was powerless. I sat for around thirty minutes in the driver's seat until the way became clear. The ambulances left in great haste, leaving the police officers to make sure the traffic began flowing once more.

I felt no pains in my stomach, just a twinge or two of discomfort, which occurred on the right-hand side of my stomach. A minute or so later, the discomfort had increased and by the time I parked my car on my driveway, I could barely walk to my front door. I made my way as quickly as I could to the couch, almost collapsing onto it. The pain was constant. As I lay prone and alone, I became extremely concerned. I hoped beyond hope that I had not disfigured the artwork performed within me by 'Smoky Eyes'. I made frequent visits to the bathroom to check if blood was once again leaking from me and was beyond relieved to see that it wasn't. I continued lying on the couch and three hours passed. The pain became less as I prayed to a god I didn't believe in and held on to the hope I had done no lasting damage.

The pain eventually ceased and I was able to leave the comfort of the couch. I took the decision not to drive anywhere unless I absolutely had to!

The following days passed without issue and the day of my PICC line insertion drew nearer. Another appointment with Dr Patel ensued and, due to the pain I had suffered during my 'fateful' drive, my initial chemotherapy cycle was postponed by a week, now commencing on 28th June 2016. However, my PICC line was still to be surgically inserted on 20th June.

The insertion date arrived and I attended the hospital once more. With each visit, the place became more familiar; however, as yet, the oncology department was unknown to me. This department would see numerous visits by me over the coming months and was located on the upper floor of the two-storey building.

I made my way past reception, along the right-hand corridor, up a flight of stairs, along a further corridor, passing the room where Professor Shamari had told me to 'let the air out.' I followed the large signs to the oncology department. Again, my ignorance got the better of me and the mere sight of the word 'oncology' installed a growing fear within me. I had never set foot in such a department and didn't even know what the word actually meant! (By the way, its definition is 'the study and treatment of tumours'.)

Would I see the poorly, ghostly figures of the bandana-wearing women I had often seen on the television, lying prone on their beds with various tubes inserted into them from every direction? The answer was no. There were no patients present for me to view, and a complete sense of serenity within the department. There was no hustle and bustle and it had the noise levels of your local library.

As I entered, I could see a small reception area to the right, containing around five comfy looking chairs, all of which were unoccupied. They surrounded a small table and behind the reception desk sat an attractive blonde female, casually dressed, who was talking on the office telephone. She gestured to me to sit and I did so. The chairs were positioned around a small table which was strewn with various pamphlets, left by a number of cancer charities. They offered varying types of advice, ranging from the correct food to eat to financial help to patients whilst they underwent treatment. Next to my chair, was a revolving magazine stand offering more pamphlets of advice. I didn't pick any of them up and just sat nervously quiet in my seat.

Time began ticking slowly once more as it always seemed to do during my visits. The receptionist finished her conversation. As she did so, I rose and made my way to her desk, informing her that I had an appointment to have my PICC line inserted. The receptionist then picked up the telephone and spoke softly to the recipient of her call, stating that I had arrived, before once more inviting me to sit.

A few minutes later, a lady dressed in dark blue nurses' overalls, black tights and black short-heeled shoes entered the reception. She was in her mid-to-late thirties and she introduced herself politely as Katherine, the lady I had spoken to previously via the telephone. Immediately I was at ease. We sat and chatted politely for a few minutes about non-cancer related matters and I immediately warmed to her. She was professional and caring in the same instance and I was confident I was safe in her hands, right from our first meeting.

She explained that the PICC line insertion would be a very simple, minor operation and that I would feel very little discomfort. The procedure would take around forty-five minutes and was to be undertaken by a gentleman called Dr Cosford. A local anaesthetic would be administered if required, but there really was no necessity for this as the procedure would cause very little discomfort anyway. She then presented me with my own pamphlet. It was the size of a small paperback book but much thinner. It contained about fifty pages and was entitled 'Your Chemotherapy Record.' It had a red cover on which a white sticker was displayed. This sticker read 'This patient is on Cytoxic Chemotherapy' and that the patient, who was me, should contact the hospital urgently if they felt unwell or displayed any of the following symptoms:

- Chest pain or difficulty in breathing
- Temperature greater than 38 degrees C (100 degrees Fahrenheit) or less than 36 degrees Celsius.
- Shivering episodes.
- Flu-like symptoms.
- Gum/nose bleeds or unusual bruising.
- Mouth ulcers that stop you eating or drinking.
- Vomiting.
- Four or more bowel movements a day or diarrhoea.

My anxiety levels rose once more!

Katherine explained to me that following chemotherapy I was more at risk of developing an infection seven to ten days after treatment and that I should wash my hands regularly. I was to use my common sense, managing the risks involved, for example avoiding someone who was coughing or sneezing. Something I would have adhered to anyway! If I used my discretion, such as not visiting crowded places during my most at-risk times, all should be well.

She further pointed out that I should not undertake any gardening whatsoever whilst I was undergoing treatment as if I were to cut myself I risked an infection. I was to avoid soft cheeses, undercooked eggs and raw fish. I was not allowed any takeaway food of any description whilst under treatment due to the way the food was reheated. Bugger, I thought to myself; no Indian or Chinese takeaways for at least six months!

After eating, I was to clean my teeth and use a mouthwash to minimise the risk of infections in my mouth. She also pointed out that I may suffer a metallic taste in my mouth following chemotherapy, which would last an undefined period of time.

Katherine further advised that when using the toilet, I should flush twice to wash away any lingering chemicals and that my dirty laundry should be stored and washed separately. Furthermore, I was to use a separate towel to anyone else in my household.

Following her information and explanations, Katherine began filling in the first two pages of my little red book. On the first page, she wrote my emergency details, my name, address and date of birth, and on the second she wrote my diagnosis and treatment. The second page read:

- Diagnosis and date: C A Rectum
- Treatment Plan: 2 Weekly
- Length of Treatment: 12 Cycles Over 6 Months
- Oncologist/Haematologist: Dr Patel
- Drug Allergies: Nil Known
- Planned Start Date: 28/6/2016

Having filled out the relevant details, Katherine said her goodbyes, telling me she would see me in just over a week and that a nurse would be along shortly to take me to see Dr Cosford, 'the PICC man'.

Whilst alone, I began thumbing through my little red book. It explained how to assess any side-effects I suffered, how to reduce the risk of infection, which foods to avoid, and to wash salads and fruits thoroughly before eating. Fruit needed peeling before being consumed and, should I develop an infection, I needed antibiotics within an hour or I could become seriously ill. I further learnt that other than the obvious sickness and lethargy symptoms, I could suffer from shingles and cold sores, and also that chemotherapy could reduce fertility, especially in men, and could make people infertile temporarily or permanently. I was to avoid sunbathing and only drink small amounts of alcohol, if any at all. No takeaways and no alcohol! Bang went my weekends!

As I continued reading from my little red book, I was interrupted by a lady wearing a light blue overall. She was around sixty years of age, with brown, curly hair which sported grey flecks. She introduced herself as Louise and asked how I was, adding the words 'my cherub' to the end of her question. We spoke politely, sharing some humour, before she led me away from the department to see 'the PICC man'.

Like Katherine, warmth and caring shone from Louise. She must have led countless people along the corridor to the room where the PICC lines were fitted, but she chatted away gleefully and, seeing that I was somewhat apprehensive regarding my looming insertion, reassured me with her comforting words.

I entered a small room and met Dr Cosford. He explained the insertion procedure to me and I was offered a local anaesthetic which I declined. I was invited to lie on the bed with my right arm extended and the procedure began. The narrow tube was inserted into the main vein on the inside of my arm, just above my elbow and just below my right bicep. It was almost a painless procedure, with the 'small scratch' into the vein being the only discomfort I felt. The doctor watched the line's progress on a small screen and I could see he was concentrating intently on its path. The line edged ever closer to my heart, finding its resting place some thirty to forty minutes later.

A cannula was fitted to the protruding end of the line and secured in place by being clipped into an adhesive patch which was then firmly stuck in place against my skin, a few inches above the inside of my right elbow. Approximately five-inches of Tubigrip, the type sportsmen and women wear to stop themselves grazing their arms, was cut and I placed my hand into it before it was pulled up my arm until it covered my new 'fitting'.

It was a painless procedure; the only discomfort came from being unable to bend my arm fully, as the device stopped me from doing so.

Dr Cosford informed me that the PICC line would now stay in place for the duration of my treatment, allowing blood to be taken and medicines received through it. This made the need for countless injections into my arm obsolete. The line would be flushed, in other words, cleaned at least once a week with a saline solution, reducing the chance of infection.

So, with the Tubigrip covering my new fitting, I left the room. Louise was waiting for me and led me back to oncology. By the time the short journey to the department was over, the area around my right elbow was somewhat red in colour. Louise removed the Tubigrip and a second opinion was requested from another nurse called Sarah.

'You're a sensitive soul,' Sarah remarked and, after a small amount of blood was taken from the PICC line, Louise advised me to contact my GP to obtain a prescription for some cream which I could apply to reduce the reaction I suffered. The nurses were not worried by what they saw, so nor was I.

It seemed that from the medical staff I had met, be it the surgeon or the nurses, any problems, minor or major, had a solution which was very reassuring.

I left the hospital, telephoning the GP's surgery on my way home. I explained why I needed the particular type of cream I had been asked to obtain and I was assured the prescription would be ready by the time I arrived. I collected the prescription, visited the nearest pharmacy, obtained and applied the cream, which had the desired effect and my very minor drama was over.

The following day, I attended the hospital and met with Louise. She duly changed my dressing, flushed out my line and again reassured me regarding my upcoming treatment. A meeting with Dr Patel followed in which he confirmed both my red and white blood cell levels were fine and confirmed my chemotherapy would begin on 28th June, some seven weeks after my surgery. A further appointment was made to see Dr Patel on 5th July, a week after my initial cycle. He explained that the appointment would be at 19:00 as he worked at the general hospital during the day, seeing his private patients in the evening. I remember thinking that these guys really do put in a full shift!

As my impending first day of treatment grew ever closer, I was naturally becoming more apprehensive. I had no idea how my body would react to the poison that would be pumped into my body, travelling swiftly through my new line into my bloodstream, before being pumped around the rest of my body, into my organs, my limbs, my torso and my brain. Would I suffer severe side-effects, average side-effects or no side-effects? I had been informed the latter was extremely unlikely but no one knew how I would react. The cells in my body were to be poisoned by the chemicals entering me and the hope was that the 'good' cells would recover and grow back healthily once more and the 'bad' cells, those that were possibly infected, would be destroyed completely, unable to re-emerge. There was no definitive answer. It was hoped the treatment would work but there simply was no guarantee. The poison and, that is what it is, would flow to every part of my being, hopefully working its magic on any 'bad' cells, sending them into oblivion, unable to return.

Of course, all this was an immense worry for my family, friends and loved ones, but what choice was there? I would be the one enduring the poisoning and all the possible terrible side-effects that could follow, but those close to me would, undoubtedly, endure their own individual side-effects. My wife and son would have to live with me and my mood swings as my mood lowered. They would see the effects of the chemicals on me. Those close to me would hear about these effects via telephone calls and visits but would probably not see me in my darkest times. I knew these times were now close and would inevitably occur. Again, although I would be the patient undergoing the treatment, I felt that somehow the sufferings of those close to me could be as serious as my sufferings. That may seem a peculiar statement to make, but that was how I felt. After all, I was in control of what I would relay to them and of course I would protect them as best I could but they would have their own thoughts and their own fears about what I was going through. No matter what I would tell them, those fears would endure. I would reassure them that I was fine and felt good; however, no matter how I expressed myself to them, they would have their doubts. Mr C had cast 'His' net far and wide.

From my experiences so far, I knew that I would be looked after by those attending to me. They would show their kindness and love, along with their professionalism. From the very first visit to my own GP, through surgery and my subsequent recovery, this had been the case, with the one exception of the painful enema experience hours before my operation. Carlos' clumsiness had been nothing more than an honest mistake and no lasting damage had been done. We, as humans, do make mistakes and as long as we learn from them, that's fine. As long as the long-term effects of those mistakes are small, that is acceptable. However, having said that, should I have any further enemas, I will check the nurse's name badge from a very safe distance!

The next few days passed without incident. Liaisons between me and the insurers occurred and all was fine. Treatment was to begin in a few days and, all being well, would continue almost until Christmas. Following the Christmas holidays, I would have a further CT scan which, I hoped, would show nothing untoward and my personal cancer experience would have passed. That was my hope, the hope of my loved ones and the hopes of the medical professionals. Only time would tell.

I had already virtually written off the year 2016. It was, without doubt, the worst year of my life – Mr C had seen to that. I knew I faced a long summer ahead of me, which would pass slowly. I would be unable to do the things I liked, such as eating out, enjoying hobbies, sunbathing, swimming and gardening. I hadn't entertained the thought of travelling to sunnier climes, enjoying foreign warm seas or the sandy beaches running alongside them. My life felt like it was on hold. However, it was a small price to pay to regain my health.

Although any thoughts of foreign travel were furthest from my mind, a holiday had been planned. A week of relaxing in the English Lake District was to take place, beginning on 29 [h] July. A log cabin on the shores of picturesque Lake Windermere was to be the destination. My wife, son, our Basset Hound and me would join my wife's sister, her husband, their two boys, their Labrador and my father-in-law. Our family had regular holidays with my wife's sister and her family (I will call them the Pendles) and we always had wonderful times together. Mr Pendle and I had, on numerous occasions, sat late into the night drinking beer and whiskey as we swapped stories, whilst putting the world to rights. This time would obviously be different as only a little alcohol would be flowing my way, but nonetheless I was looking forward to our week together. The effect of chemotherapy would be upon me by the time of the holiday but I was determined to enjoy the week. It would be a welcome relief from the numerous hospital visits which I had experienced and those due to take place. It would be a time to cherish and, hopefully, a time to leave any frightening thoughts several hundred miles behind.

It would also be an important time for my father-in-law, John, and his two girls. It had only been a few months since his beloved Jean was taken so cruelly from him and it would be the first time he and his daughters had been together for a substantial period of time, and they would be able to talk, letting their feelings flow whilst remembering their mother and wife. They would be able to share their special memories and be able to reflect together, reflecting on the good times.

We were all looking forward to the holiday and I hoped I would be able to enjoy the week, free from hospital visits and without the poison flowing through, scuppering our plans.

This thought worried me. Would I be too ill to enjoy our

holiday? What if I became ill whilst being so far from home? How would my family cope, what would be the plan? Troubled, I contacted Katherine. Once more, I had been worrying unduly. I explained my planned holiday to her, along with my worries. In that one telephone call she put me at ease. She explained that although my treatment was extremely important, so was my quality of life. If my chemotherapy cycle was scheduled for when I was on holiday, she would work around it. Should I become unwell whilst away, I was to travel to Lancaster Infirmary where I would be looked after. Katherine told me to call the emergency number which was written on the front of my little red book and whoever answered would contact her. She would then contact the Infirmary to inform them of my impending arrival so they could prepare. Ironically, it transpired that Katherine had lived near to the Infirmary and had previously worked there! It really did seem that a problem shared was, indeed, a problem halved!

Leading up to my initial cycle, two minor problems arose, both relating to my PICC line. The first was sleeping. I found that when I bent my arm, the fixing holding my cannula in place would dig into my skin and invariably wake me up. There was very little I could do about this, apart from not bending my arm. I would fall asleep with my arm outstretched only to be woken numerous times from my slumber, having unwittingly bent my arm whilst sleeping. It was beyond my control and there was nothing I could really do about it. It was something I would have to live with for at least six months and I knew I would. It wasn't a worry; after all, I was about to have numerous medicines and other liquids pumped into me which would make my uncomfortable elbow seem insignificant. It was a minor issue and didn't really affect my quality of life.

The second issue was showering. My line needed to be protected and it was imperative that it was kept dry. It needed covering whilst washing. Initially I found the answer to be some good old fashioned cling film! My wife would wrap my arm numerous times before I could shower and the plastic performed its task well, although it wasn't particularly practical. On my own, I was unable to wrap my arm adequately. I would try holding the plastic in my free hand, with my right arm outstretched; however, I failed miserably in wrapping the thin plastic tightly enough on most occasions and I was unable to offer my line the protection it deserved. As soon as I would hold my arm straight down, the plastic would start unwrapping and failure ensued. I took to holding one end of the sticky plastic in my mouth whilst attempting to wrap it around my arm with my free hand but always seemed to end up with more plastic in my mouth than around my arm!

Prior to my first cycle, I spoke to Louise whilst she was working at the hospital. She solved my showering issues immediately. She gave me the details of a company nearby who would deliver what she called a PICC line protector to my home address.

'That will solve your problems, my cherub,' she stated. She

was right.

I ordered the protector and when it arrived, my showering became a pleasure once more. The protector was a hollow plastic tube with a round malleable rubber piece at each end. I placed my arm through the top rubber, into the hollow tube and through the bottom rubber. Once in position, one rubber end sealed itself tightly around my wrist and the other tightly around my upper arm, forming a waterproof seal at each end and, hey presto, I was a happy shower-goer once more! Again, problem solved!

These may seem trivial problems and they were to me too. However, trivial problems grow into larger problems. Had I not continued to keep the end of my line dry, more serious problems would have arisen. I may have developed an infection so my line would have been removed and a new one inserted. With an infection, my treatment would be halted until it was safe to start it again. I was about to face various problems regarding my treatment and I certainly didn't want an infectious PICC line to go with them.

Louise had told me that in all her years of experience she had only seen a few PICC line issues. On one occasion a patient arrived at the oncology department for his treatment, holding his whole line in the palm of his hand! Somehow, he had removed it or, someone had removed it for him.

'Why the hell would you do that'? I asked.

Louise explained that he claimed he had caught the end of it on something without realising and accidentally pulled the whole length of it out of his arm!

'Naturally,' Louise said humorously, 'he didn't undergo treatment on that day.'

She told me of another patient who was a keen rugby player. Despite having the line and undergoing treatment, he played rugby each Saturday, without fail. Louise and the nurses did not recommend this course of action and often expected him to attend for treatment with a damaged or non-existent line, but, amazingly, their fears were never realised. He didn't miss any treatments, no damage occurred and, as far as she knew, he was now fit and healthy.

'You see, my cherub, even with treatment, your life goes on.'

Despite what she told me, I decided not to start playing rugby!

CHAPTER NINE

Poisoned

Twenty-eighth of June 2016. My day of reckoning had arrived. My first cycle of chemotherapy was imminent and I was filled with trepidation. I was a 'chemo virgin' and my 'deflowering' was about to take place. My thoughts on this day were slightly peculiar. I was nervous, apprehensive, worried, fearful and ignorant of what was about to take place. However, I was also slightly excited. I looked on the next stage of this journey as something of an adventure. I would be exploring the unknown, taking steps along a new path and discovering new experiences. I knew that many of those experiences would be difficult to endure, but surely there would be some pleasantness on this journey, wouldn't there? After all, I was to be attended to, almost pampered, by those looking after me. I was their patient and the focus of their working day would be on me. Who doesn't like a bit of pampering? Who doesn't like the attention of professionals being directed their way? I would meet and get to know new people, learn from them, accept their advice and, hopefully, become important to them. I was to be attended to by caring professionals and, yes, I was slightly excited, although my excitement most certainly did not outweigh my apprehension and fears.

No one knew what side-effects would present themselves – how could they? I had never been through this treatment before and I would probably react differently to other patients as we are all different, especially when it comes to chemotherapy. I had been told what *could* happen but no one knew what *would* happen. That, alone, instilled just a little excitement within me. It was now time to see. I clung to the thought that my side-effects would be minimal. Perhaps I wouldn't feel too ill or not be overcome by fatigue. Perhaps life would be almost normal, with little change, other than the regular hospital visits I would experience over the following six months. The only thing left now was to wait and see. That was all I could do. Undergo my first cycle, do as instructed and wait.

I arrived at the hospital in good time for my 09:00 appointment. I made my way to the oncology department, clutching my little red book tightly in my hand. My wife accompanied me and we met with Katherine and Louise. After the preliminaries were recorded, which included my blood pressure, heart rate, temperature, height and weight, we were led along the corridor to a small room. There were approximately six private rooms on each side of the narrow corridor and mine was the fifth room along on the right-hand side. The room was pleasant and the summer sunshine was beating through the large oblong window at the rear of the room. In the room was a single bed, an armchair, a standing lamp, a sideboard on which stood a medium-sized television, a small coffee table and two dining room chairs. The room had an en suite toilet, a basin and a shower cubicle.

As we waited, I stared out of the window at the lush grounds surrounding the hospital and the neatly cut grass and trimmed bushes. Suddenly, there it was once more. The resident peacock, in all its splendour, was roaming the lawns, seemingly without a care in the world. I beckoned my wife to the window. We watched the peacock for several minutes as it meandered its way across the grass, before it turned a corner, disappearing from view and no doubt continuing its carefree business.

Moments later Louise entered the room, accompanied by another nurse who introduced herself as Fiona. Both were dressed in light-blue overalls and Louise was pulling a mobile drip stand alongside her. A small plastic bag, filled with a clear liquid, was hanging limply from it. She was carrying several narrow, transparent plastic bags with her, which contained the thin tubes to be attached to the bag hanging from the drip stand. In turn, these tubes would be attached from the bag to the mechanical dispenser, situated approximately half-way down the drip stand and into the cannula at the end of my PICC line.

Louise took the tubes from the sterile packaging and fitted them into position before setting the dispenser to the correct setting. Various buttons on the dispenser were pushed and the liquid began flowing. The liquid felt cold as it entered my arm but, as it entered my bloodstream, the coolness disappeared and I felt nothing.

Louise and Fiona explained that, initially, antihistamines, steroids and anti-sickness drugs would be pumped into my body before my FOLFOX treatment, which comprised folinic acid, oxaliplatin and fluorouracil (5 FU), began.

Only a small amount of fluorouracil was to be introduced into my system via the drip. The main body of this treatment would enter my body via a pump which would be attached to my PICC line before I left. I would then wear this pump for two further days, and, over forty-six hours, the remaining fluorouracil I needed would be pumped into me.

Both nurses reassured me and told me that if I had any questions they would answer them. Both their caring and professionalism again shone through and I was confident I was in safe hands. Before leaving the room, they told me they would return to check on me shortly. Should I need them, I was to use the 'call' button which was attached to the bed by a long thin plastic tube housing its wires.

So, I sat in the armchair and my wife lay on the bed, as the cold liquid filled my bloodstream and made its way around my body. My eyes became transfixed on the bag of clear liquid hanging from the drip stand as its contents entered into me. It dripped, very slowly, filling the tube, and I became resigned to the fact that this day was going to pass extremely slowly, only interrupted by the nurses entering the room to remove the empty plastic bags and replace them with full ones.

It took around ninety minutes for the anti-sickness, steroids and antihistamines to drip into me before the

FOLFOX regime began. During those ninety minutes, two things occurred. Firstly, I began urinating almost every thirty minutes or so. With each trip to the toilet, I slowly and nervously pulled the drip stand with me, praying I wouldn't somehow manage to tip it over or dislodge the tube. Each visit and return became a chore in itself as I ponderously pulled the stand and its attachments alongside me.

Secondly, and more embarrassingly, I began passing large amounts of wind. Every minute or so, wind would be expelled rapidly from my nether regions and along with the expulsion came the inevitable stench – and it was a real stench!

My wife continually asked me how I was feeling and I answered her reassuringly on each occasion. I was truthful in my answers as I was actually feeling fine during the initial process.

She turned on the television and we sat watching various repeats of various programmes along with the news channels. These tele-visual treats did not help the day pass any quicker!

Then it was time for the FOLFOX regime to begin. Firstly, the folinic acid entered my body, followed by the oxaliplatin and then the small amount of fluorouracil entered my system. The next stage of this journey had now well and truly begun. I had no real fears whilst these liquids entered my system although I feared how they would affect my body over the coming days.

I barely felt anything whilst they entered me and the worst thing really was the boredom as I sat waiting for each plastic bag to empty but empty they did, albeit very slowly. The bag emptying process took around five hours before Louise produced the pump containing the remaining fluorouracil which I was to wear for the next two days.

The pump was the size and shape of an average-sized soft drink can. It was made of a clear, strong plastic with a flat, pink, plastic 'ring' at the top. This 'ring' was about an inch thick and was tapered towards its top. Protruding from the tapered top was a small plastic cylinder which was about half an inch in height and width, from which ran a thin plastic tube.

Inside the main body of the pump, I could see what I would describe as a small inflated balloon, which almost filled the whole of the inside of the pump. The thin plastic tube running from the top of the pump was then fitted to the cannula on the inside of my elbow and the rest of the fluorouracil began its slow journey into my system.

Louise advised me on my 'wearing' of the pump.

'Do you have a bum bag, my cherub?' she politely inquired. I racked my brain as this was something I'd only ever taken on summer holidays and had rarely even worn.

'Yes,' was my reply.

Louise clearly wasn't too confident in my reply and turned to my wife. 'When you find it, use it to carry the pump,' she continued.

My wife nodded and smiled at Louise.

Great, I thought to myself. Not only did I have a pump

attached to me with its long thin tube impossible to disguise, I'd have to wear a bum bag for the next two days! Should I venture to the local supermarket, I couldn't help wondering what people would think! No doubt some would be bemused by the sight of a fellow shopper complete with a bum bag and a tube coming from it, running up my arm. Some may well have viewed me as a very unambitious suicide bomber! Again, it was what it was and a time for others to now be the ignorant ones.

Before I was able to leave the hospital, Fiona appeared carrying a paper bag which she placed on the bed. The bag contained an abundance of tablets to aid my recovery. Over the next few days, I would be required to take a grand total of nine tablets each day, mainly to reduce any nausea I was likely to suffer. At least I wouldn't go hungry!

More advice followed. The nurses reiterated that I needed to clean my teeth after eating, along with using the strong mouth wash which had been prescribed and was amongst the tablets in the paper bag. I was to check my pump regularly and should be able to see the balloon within it slowly deflating. Another tip was to weigh the pump on my kitchen scales at regular intervals to make sure it was getting lighter as the liquid entered my body. If I had any concerns, I was to contact the department immediately and any necessary arrangements would be made.

An appointment was made for me to return in two days for my pump removal. All this information was recorded in my little red book and farewells were exchanged. My wife and

I thanked the nurses and we left. My little red book was in one hand and I carried my pump in the other.

Immediately our short journey home began, I felt very insecure. For the past five hours or so I had had the security of the nurses. One push of the call button and a nurse would come to my aid. Whilst at the hospital, any problems would be dealt with almost immediately, with the expertise of the medical team. Now, things were very different. I would be 'home alone.' Yes, of course, my wife and son were close by. However, they had no medical training. Should some abnormality occur, should I bother the hospital? No one knew what side-effects I would suffer. No one could tell me with any certainty that tomorrow I wouldn't vomit or have diarrhoea, or that the largest ulcer known to man wouldn't grow in my mouth. No one knew. It was a waiting game. This or that might occur or it may not. My body might react like this or it might not. Should problems arise, they would be dealt with, but they couldn't be halted before they arose because no one, including myself, knew what those problems would be.

Again, my ignorance began breeding fear as had so often been the case on this journey. I felt completely helpless during the hours after my treatment. I checked my appearance in the mirror and placed the thermometer against my forehead countless times. Nothing happened. I had not grown an extra ear and my nose remained its normal size and shape. My temperature remained stable. I could do nothing but wait. I knew the chemicals and medicines would affect me in some way, but when and how? I waited, feeling the nervousness a driver feels when he or she takes off their 'L' plates and heads out on the open road, alone, for the first time. Nervousness, apprehension and fear all came at once. Again my rollercoaster was on its travels, gaining momentum.

Time passed slowly that evening. I watched television but took in little information. My wife and I chatted about the day's events and how well I had been looked after by the nurses. I knew they would become a major part of my life in the coming six months, along with Dr Patel, the oncologist. I felt I was in safe hands.

My wife and I chatted then went into the kitchen. It was good to talk, taking my mind briefly away from the worries in my mind. I was concentrating now on our chatting, so much so that I forgot one piece of very important advice I had been given. The fridge was close by and I was feeling peckish. Instinctively, I opened the fridge and peeked inside to see what I could nibble on whilst waiting for dinner. One of my favourite nibbles was staring back at me, all alone, on a white ceramic plate. A single, homemade sausage roll, almost pleading with me to reach in and grab it.

Before I could do so, I felt my wife's hand on my shoulder, pulling me back.

'What are you doing, you idiot?' she questioned, scornfully.

I looked at her, utterly dumbfounded and completely innocently, in a state of shock.

'I'm just getting a sausage roll,' I replied indignantly.

As soon as I had replied, the penny dropped. I had come so close to reaching into the cold fridge with my unprotected fingers, something I had been warned against doing.

'Has that stuff already affected your brain?' my wife jokingly questioned. She removed the plate from the fridge and ordered me not to touch it until she'd warmed the roll.

I was about to tell her to stop fussing, when I realised she wasn't. She was protecting me, looking after me, not wanting me to suffer any avoidable pain. With the snack suitably warmed, I was able to tuck in, and tuck in I most certainly did! I immediately wished I hadn't. I took a large bite and chewed. A searing pain erupted at the back of my mouth. It was the type of pain that makes you shout out loudly, taking your breath away. It was almost on a level comparable to when Carlos was unable to find his target on the day of my surgery. The pain was at the rear of my lower jaw, on both sides, and I immediately stopped chewing just for a second. I then opened my jaw very slightly before closing it and repeated the motion very quickly. The pain continued with each chew, but the smaller the chew, the less the pain. After around five of these small but rapid chews the pain ceased, allowing me to chew normally.

I must have looked a sad, almost comical sight, standing there in the kitchen, bum bag around my waist, a plastic tube running from the bum bag, up my arm and under my protective Tubigrip, shouting loudly whilst eating a sausage roll!

So, I had experienced my first chemotherapy side effect. It was a painful experience and, in all my wildest dreams, I never thought it would involve a single, humble, little homemade sausage roll. My wife had 'saved' me from the refrigerator, but the sausage roll had bitten back! How surreal this was all becoming.

The main meal of the evening was consumed, again with my initial chews causing pain. My chewing technique helped control it and I saw myself as resembling a mouse eating a piece of cheese, chewing quickly, but barely opening its mouth.

I followed the advice I had been given by those who knew best, diligently cleaning my teeth and rinsing my mouth with the mouthwash I had been supplied with. I flushed the toilet twice after use and showered with my pump tightly wrapped in cling film whilst my PICC line was covered by its protector. I dried myself with my appointed towel and kept my worn clothes separate, ready for washing.

During the evening, no further dramas occurred. As often occurs at these times, my wife 'posted' a photograph she had taken during my initial cycle on one of the social media sites, tagging me in it. Both of us were not avid users of social media and rarely posted anything. Whenever we did post, we received nominal amounts of likes or comments and would feel proud if even five people showed interest.

Within a few hours, we had received thirty-three comments and a similar amount of likes regarding the photograph. Now, to you avid users of these platforms, these figures may seem pretty pathetic, but to us they were massive! People I knew well, along with those I barely knew, were commenting and liking the post. Some very kind comments were made, all giving me hope and support. People from around the globe, as far apart as Sweden, Australia and the UK, took the time to look, read and comment on my plight. These comments and likes meant so much to both of us, more than anyone could ever know.

Another act of kindness also took place around this time. A lovely lady I worked with undertook a charity run, raising money to help the fight against Mr C. I dare say it had been many years since she had run any significant distance and I'm sure the run was a real struggle, but she completed it. Some of her friends and family joined her and their efforts raised hundreds of pounds for the charity. She sent me a photograph of herself dressed in her running kit, complete with my name emblazoned on the back of her top. For the first time since cancer had called upon me, tears filled my eyes. As I told her, those tears were not of pain or sorrow, but of happiness; they were 'good' tears. It shows the effect a cancer diagnosis and the subsequent treatment can have. You see, as I have said previously, cancer casts its web far and wide, affecting so many.

The evening passed, slowly turning to night. Physically, I felt fine. My wife had shown me the love and support I needed and had done so since the beginning of my journey.

Around 22:00 we went to bed. Sleeping was a problem. I

was slowly getting used to the uncomfortable PICC line and now I had to wear a bum bag. I could only lie on my back and each time I rolled to the right, the pump dug into me. I worried that, somehow, I would catch the tube running from the pump into my arm and dislodge it. Unable to sleep, my mind began racing. What would the following day bring? How would I feel? What would I look like? These questions were not answerable, at least not yet. Only time would tell.

After a few hours sleep, night turned to day. When I awoke, I felt completely different to the previous day. The liquids that had been and were being pumped into me began to take their toll. I felt extremely sick and the colour had drained from my face. I was tired and felt weak.

I consumed the tablets as prescribed, in the hope they would cure my nausea. They didn't. The feelings of sickness persisted along with the pain in my jaw when I took the first bites of any food. My wife and son left for work and college respectively, and I was left alone to rest. I dozed on the couch for only minutes at a time, before the overwhelming feelings of sickness woke me. I visited the bathroom on numerous occasions, always thinking I would vomit, but I didn't. That was my day. The nausea didn't subside. It remained at the same level, neither reducing nor increasing.

I checked my temperature hourly, took my tablets, cleaned my teeth, used the mouthwash and lay on the couch, bum bag constantly attached. Whenever I took anything from the refrigerator, I used a tea towel for protection. The day seemed one of the longest I'd ever experienced, broken by only short bouts of sleep. I looked and felt extremely ill and wished the nausea away, but the wishing didn't help. Nothing changed throughout the day. As the time for bed approached, something else happened: I began to hiccup. Now, having the hiccups sounds pretty trivial I grant you but these particular hiccups felt like they had been sent to me from the very depths of hell. They seemed to come from deep within my body and my whole chest rose with each one that left my mouth. They were deep and painful and continued for over two hours. By the time they'd passed, my whole chest ached. Of course I had experienced hiccups before, just like everyone has, but never like these.

Finally, with their passing, I managed to fall asleep. My chest hurt and I felt sick and weak. I was wearing my bum bag which housed my pump, uncomfortable in itself, but I knew that the following day it would be removed. The balloon within it was slowly deflating as the 'medicine' entered my body. I was looking forward to its removal and hoped its removal would be the beginning of the end of my nausea.

At 01:30 the next morning, my hiccups returned with similar severity. Again, they lasted around two hours and again my chest ached with every deep movement as the air was expelled from my mouth. Once they passed, they left my chest slowly recovering from the pain they had caused. I was unable to sleep for any length of time, mainly due to the nausea I was experiencing. I would sleep for maybe an hour before waking for two and then 'grabbing' another hour. The day had been long, but the night was even longer.

The following day eventually came with no changes to the way I was feeling. I attended the hospital and Louise disconnected my now empty pump. I explained my issues to her, from the hiccups to my feelings of sickness. She was not shocked by what I told her as she had seen these effects in patients before. She told me they would pass and was sympathetic to my plight. She suggested I eat something containing ginger as that may ease my nausea, along with getting an anti-sickness wrist band. She added that although neither of these had been scientifically proven, a number of patients had previously told her they had helped. I told her I was willing to try anything and would take her advice.

Louise then flushed my line and further appointments were made. The first was 5th July for a further flushing and the second was 11th July (the day before my second cycle) for a blood test and flushing.

With that, I left the hospital, clutching my little red book in one hand and my bum bag in the other. I was pump-free, at least until my next treatment, which made me slightly more upbeat.

From the hospital, I travelled directly to my local supermarket. I purchased two packets of ginger flavoured biscuits and two anti-sickness wrist bands. I returned to my car and devoured a packet of the biscuits and put a wristband on each wrist. I headed home where I ate the second packet of biscuits and assumed my position on the couch, and waited and waited. Hours passed without change. For some these tips may have worked, but for me, I noticed no change.

My nausea continued and the colour didn't return to my face.

That night, during the small hours, I awoke once more, although this was not due to 'the mother of all hiccups'. I would just open my eyes and wake up. I couldn't sleep and found myself feeling very hungry and sick, both at the same time. I would get up, take my anti-sickness pills and watch a film, constantly hoping I would feel better. I was so hungry I could have cooked and eaten a whole, large pizza, then easily cooked another and eaten that.

I put this hunger down to the steroids I was taking orally and which had been pumped into me. One of the tablets I was taking was Dexamethasone. This is a steroid which has been prescribed for many years, but since the Covid 19 pandemic struck, it has been mentioned on numerous news channels. I'm sure if it's good enough for Mr Donald Trump, then it's good enough for me!

I knew that if I submitted to my pangs of hunger, I could easily gain a large amount of weight, so I fought against what my brain was telling me. I made sure I cooked chicken breasts, along with some healthy fish, in the hope that would cure my cravings and I would not experience a huge weight gain.

Friday 1st July 2016 arrived and it was now three days since my first cycle. I continued feeling sick and my doses of anti-sickness medicine and packets of ginger biscuits seemed ineffective. My temperature, thankfully, remained stable. I still suffered the pain in my jaw when eating and still took care when retrieving foods and liquids from the refrigerator. The tea towel was becoming a close friend! I was not willing to chance removing items from the fridge without the trusty tea towel because the pain in my jaw was continuing and, I surmised, that my finger tips would mirror similar pain. I could protect my fingers, but it was almost impossible to do the same to my jaw. The pain in my jaw constantly reminded me that the liquids that had been pumped into me were flowing through my system, weaving their own kind of 'magic.'

I continued cleaning my teeth after eating and it was something I was now getting used to. My teeth were almost sparkling and were clearly, other than following a visit to the dental hygienist, the cleanest they'd ever been!

I began to notice other small changes to my body and its functions. I had not opened my bowels since the morning of my first cycle which was highly unusual. I was normally very regular, definitely a 'one a day man' but it had now been three days. I didn't even feel the slightest urge so I began taking laxatives, the kind you can buy off the shelf. I waited, but nothing. As it had only been three days, I wasn't too worried so I continued with the laxatives and waited patiently.

Friday became Saturday. I woke during the early hours and took my normal position on the couch, taking in the 02:00 matinee. I continued feeling sick so an anti-sickness tablet followed my devouring of two chicken breasts and a tin of tuna. Movie completed, I made a quick temperature check and back to bed I went. Sleeping was difficult but eventually I managed it. I would drift off to sleep, only to be awakened as I rolled onto my right side and the attachments on my line dug into me, waking me once more.

Sunday followed. Again, the early matinee, anti-sickness medicine and a small feast took place before more sleep was attempted. I awoke around 10:00 and decided that on this day, some five days after chemotherapy, that I would open my bowels. It was now a worry. Other than the period following surgery, I had not suffered from constipation. However, during that period I had eaten very little. Things were now very different. Despite feeling constantly sick, I had eaten well since chemo but despite food entering my body, nothing solid had exited.

I got up, had an anti-sickness tablet along with a strong coffee, hoping that the latter would help with my impending trip to the toilet. Coffee consumed, I visited the bathroom. I sat, waited, pushed, stood up and sat down numerous times and pushed some more. Nothing! I continued standing, sitting pushing and waiting. I repeated these motions numerous times, all to no avail. I began to lose hope when, hallelujah, something stirred within me. I pushed and pushed and could feel something was definitely on its way. Whatever it was felt extremely solid and I forced a small part of it out of me. However, nothing fell into the still water below. Again I pushed with all my might, moving the 'object' very slightly, before I almost gave up once more. I knew I was unable to give up now as I had reached 'the point of no return'. Something very dense was slowly leaving me but still no ripples appeared below. Stopping my efforts now was impossible, so they continued in the hope that whatever it was that had partly left me would continue its journey. It was as though I was trying to pass the proverbial brick with a corner of it out but the rest of it very much within me.

By this stage, things were extremely uncomfortable and were rapidly becoming painful. Push by push, millimetre by millimetre, my 'brick' was shifting. I was now experiencing such discomfort that I left my sitting position and found myself crawling around on my hands and knees behind the locked bathroom door. I had never experienced this discomfort before and it was rendering me helpless. I must have looked a pathetic sight, crawling around naked on the bathroom floor, huffing and puffing, just wishing I could have a shit!

Some ninety minutes later, yes, you read that correctly, ninety minutes later, having managed to resume my seated position, my 'brick' was ejected, followed by countless other 'bricks.' They all splashed loudly into the water. These 'bricks' were so dense and so numerous they began to build from the bottom of the ceramic bowl, covering the water and protruding from its surface. I had managed to block the toilet without using any toilet paper whatsoever!

After several flushings, the bricks were eventually broken and they continued their journeys deep into the sewerage system. They had left me exhausted and I walked gingerly back to bed.

I had been on this earth forty-nine years and could only remember experiencing constipation twice, both of which had occurred within the last two months. The latter was much, much worse and it is something I whole-heartedly do not recommend.

Monday came with me waking around 04:00 but managing to get back to sleep within half an hour or so. I also noticed that my feelings of sickness were not so strong. I took my three anti-sickness tablets at regular intervals and dozed on the couch whenever possible.

On this day, the sixth day after my chemotherapy, I decided to try something new. I plucked up the necessary courage to take something from the refrigerator without the use of any PPE. In trepidation, I opened the fridge and quickly looked inside. The plastic milk bottle was upright, resting in the door shelf. With my left hand, I reached into the coldness, grabbing the milk bottle by its handle, and pulled it as fast as I could from its resting place. I quickly placed it on the kitchen work surface. I felt no pain in my fingers and made my coffee before lifting the milk bottle once more. I unscrewed the green, plastic cap and added the white liquid to my drink. No pain or discomfort occurred and this small action, which would be automatic for so many, along with the fact I didn't feel so sick, made this day a good day!

That night, I slept through. My sleep was only broken by me rolling onto my right side and my 'fitting' digging into me. Things were definitely improving. It had taken six long days to reach this point but it had arrived, just as I had been told it would. The last six days had been a real struggle. My hiccups from hell had occurred on two days and the pain in my jaw, when eating, had lasted for three days. My constant feelings of sickness had continued for five days before they began to reduce and my nightly waking and constant hunger had now stopped.

It was now 5th July 2016, a week after my initial cycle. Although I was still feeling sick, the feelings were not so strong or as constant. Their severity was definitely weaker and I set off to the hospital to have my PICC line flushed, following which I explained my toilet problems to Louise; she explained that was a common side effect following treatment. I was prescribed a strong laxative along with more anti-sickness tablets, returned home and awaited my evening appointment with Dr Patel.

The day passed peacefully and evening came. I was accompanied to my appointment by my wife and my little red book. We entered the hospital and I checked in at reception before we both sat on one of the comfortable chairs.

As we waited, a peculiar thought crossed my mind. I could see no one else clutching little red books. People were sat with crutches by their sides, or limping as they visited the nearby toilet. Some were holding an arm across their chest, with the aid of a sling, but there was no sign of any red books. Surely Dr Patel had not interrupted his evening just on my behalf. Suddenly, I felt peculiarly important! These patients clearly had problems, their own health issues, which were of great importance to them, but surely their issues were not as serious as mine. They weren't undergoing the dreaded chemo. I was, and the last seven days had really affected me. With these thoughts, I placed my little red book on my lap, with its title displayed in bold white letters facing up. I thought, 'You lot with your dodgy hips, sore feet or frozen shoulders, check me out, I've got cancer!' It was as though in the pecking order of illnesses, I was at the top. I was peculiarly proud of this. Perhaps, subconsciously or consciously, I was looking for a little sympathy after what I had been through over the last seven days. Cancer certainly does peculiar things, not only to your body but also to your mind.

Dr Patel appeared from the corridor. Our eyes met, no words were needed. My wife and I rose and followed him into his office. We sat opposite him and he asked how I had felt since my first cycle. I explained everything to him, the feeling of sickness, the hiccups, the jaw pain, the sleeplessness, hunger pangs and the constipation, 'the whole nine yards'. He was unmoved. Clearly, he had seen these side-effects before! His lack of surprise was reassuring and I questioned him on several issues. Answering me honestly, he informed me that with each cycle I received, I would become slightly weaker each time. Each therapy would have a cumulative effect, each one weakening me slightly more than the last. This was not good news. I had felt like death warmed up following my first cycle and the good doctor was now informing me that things were going to get worse! My body would suffer more with each treatment and I couldn't help wondering what I would feel like after twelve cycles, let alone two or three! I was frightened and it clearly showed. Dr Patel read my mind.

'Anthony,' he began, 'your treatment is extremely important and it is also very important that the treatment is completed.'

My heart sank.

'But so is your quality of life and I, along with the nurses, will do all we can to make sure that quality is the best it can be,' he continued.

Although I felt and very clearly looked ill, these words gave me hope. At this point in my life, my rollercoaster was plummeting faster than ever before but at Dr Patel's words it applied its brakes ever so slightly. It certainly wasn't on an upward curve yet, that was a long way off, but I felt like my foot had moved from its accelerator, just covering its brakes.

I questioned the doctor further. Even by now, I had little knowledge of what cancer actually was and what caused it. He was happy to answer, confirming that tumours were caused by cells multiplying, growing rapidly, becoming out of control and leading to their growth, and that the reason this happens is due to a fault within our own cells which causes this multiplication. This multiplication then destroys tissues and can spread to the organs. When this occurs, the cancer is described as metastatic. I was learning more about cancer seemingly every day.

Our meeting finished and a further one was made for 19th July 2016. Basically, my life over the next six months or so was to be hospital, hospital, hospital. It was to be like this:

Week One

Monday: Bloods taken and levels checked. PICC line flushed.

Tuesday: Chemotherapy.

Thursday: Pump removal and PICC line flushed.

Week Two

Monday: Bloods taken and their levels checked. PICC line flushed.

Tuesday: Meeting with the oncologist, Dr Patel.

Then begin week one again. That was how it was, providing there were no complications, which would lead to further hospital visits.

As I left the hospital, Dr Patel's words kept repeating in my mind:

'But so is your quality of life...'

CHAPTER TEN

Two Out of Three Definitely Ain't Bad!

The Saturday following my appointment with the oncologist, my wife and I had a welcome break from what had become our normal way of life. My good friend, Patrick, and his lovely fiancée, Susan, married. The wedding ceremony took place in a small village nearby, with friends and family in attendance. I had made my mind up that no matter how I felt, I would be with them to enjoy their special day as best I could. By now my nausea was nowhere near the level it had been and, as each day had passed, it had reduced. I was still taking my anti-sickness pills as often as I was allowed and still checking my temperature constantly. I sought advice from both Katherine and Louise about whether I should attend due to my immune system being affected by the treatment. Both had said, unreservedly, that I should.

'Just avoid anyone who obviously has a cold,' they had told me.

Had their advice been different, I would have followed it, begrudgingly, but both said I needed to continue with my life as best I could.

The ceremony passed without a hitch. Patrick looked a picture in his blue, three-piece suit and his bride, although fashionably late, looked beautiful and resplendent in her wedding dress, veil and tiara.

From the church, we travelled directly to the wedding meal, held in a hall nearby. Speeches and toasts followed and it was then time for the dancing!

After performing the 'dodgy two-step' a few times, I began to feel tired. It was around 20:30 and time for me to make my excuses, although none were necessary to the happy couple. Both knew, to some extent, what I had been experiencing since my first cycle, so a hug and a handshake later and my wife and I departed, leaving the revellers to enjoy the rest of the celebrations. I wished with all my heart that I could continue partying until the early hours, but there was just no way. My body was telling me it was time to rest, so I listened, agreed and did what I was told. I slept particularly well that night, something that hadn't occurred much lately.

Sunday came and a miracle occurred! I woke around 07:00 and I didn't feel sick! Not in the slightest. It was now twelve days since my first cycle and it was only now that I felt no nausea. I was still feeling fatigued and still looked pale, but the feelings of sickness had left my body. It was a good day despite the fact that with each hour that passed, it was an hour closer to my next treatment. That was something I was now dreading. There was no sense of a little excitement anymore – that had long passed. I knew what would happen following my second appearance for chemo but I also knew that my journey had to continue. Each cycle I underwent was a cycle closer to the last, due in December, still some five months away. I wished I could close my eyes and that date would be upon me. People had always told me not to wish my life away but I truly wished away the next five months. I knew my wishes would go unanswered and that the next period of my life would be the hardest I would have to endure. I had little choice in the matter and endure it I would.

Monday came, the day before my second treatment. Another trip to the hospital to have a blood test and another flushing of my PICC line by Louise came and went. My dread of the following day continued but my dread couldn't stop time and Tuesday 12th July 2016 was soon upon me.

This time I travelled to the hospital alone. I saw no point in my wife accompanying me as all I would do for the five or six hours of being pumped with medicines and chemicals would be watch daytime television, chat to those attending to me, visit the toilet on numerous occasions, and look out of the window, hopefully spying the resident peacock as it patrolled its grounds.

By 09:30 I was attached to the drip. The cold liquids entered my body. Antihistamines, anti-sickness tablets and steroids, one after the other, were pumped slowly into me, followed by the chemicals I dreaded. Again, I was mainly attended to by Louise and Fiona. We chatted, with Louise adding 'my cherub' to the end of most of her sentences. I learnt that she loved horses and kept at least one locally. She told me about her family and I told her about mine. I could feel there was a bond being built as we chatted freely, unguardedly and honestly with each other.

It was the same with Fiona. She told me about her family and how she missed her son who was studying dance in London. He visited when he could, but as any caring mother knows, it was never enough. Fiona spoke of how she had hopes of entering palliative care, the treatment and care of those who have a life-limiting illness. She told me she wanted to make a difference to people, helping those most in need.

What shone brightly from both these individuals was their wholehearted feelings towards those they treated. Nursing was not just an occupation for them. They didn't just turn up for work to watch the clock tick around to finishing time; they actually wanted to make a patient's life better.

It was the same for all the medical staff I had met on this journey. All of them wanted to help those in need as best they could, without exception. They were just normal people, as normal as you and me, until you knew them just a little. When you did, you could see how much they cared about what they were doing and how much they wanted to help those under their care and guidance.

So, having watched enough daytime television to last me at least a week, having passed plenty of wind and urinated every half an hour or so, with pump attached and my paper bag almost full of anti-sickness pills, I left the hospital. It was now around 15:30.

That evening, I noticed a change to my body. It was a change I had been told may occur. I had a constant metallic taste inside my mouth. It was another side-effect of the treatment. It was as though I was chewing on a piece of metal. The pain to the rear of my jaw returned when I ate and I had discomfort in my fingertips when cold water from the tap touched them. Along with my metallic mouth, my lips became very dry. Thankfully my temperature remained normal and my nausea hadn't kicked in yet.

The next morning, I awoke around 04:30. I was starving and didn't feel at all like sleeping. My mouth and lips were very dry and my nausea began.

Throughout the following day, the feelings of sickness increased and the pain continued when I ate. The metallic taste in my mouth had passed by now. Day became evening and evening became night. As I lay my head on my pillow, hoping to sleep, my hiccups returned. Again they were extreme and by the time they had passed, some two hours later, my whole chest ached. I managed to sleep for a few hours before waking early, once more craving food, glorious, food!

As my mouth felt drier than the Sahara desert, I made my way to the kitchen and filled a pint glass with water, making sure the cold liquid didn't touch my finger tips. I took a large gulp. I immediately wished I hadn't! Searing pain ran through both sides of my lower jaw, making me yell out and spit the water back into the sink. So, now not only could I not eat without feeling like someone had thrust a red-hot poker into my mouth, it was painful to drink as well!

Later that day, I visited the hospital to have my pump removed. The balloon inside it had emptied its contents of fluorouracil into my system and now sat limply within the transparent walls which housed it. I told Louise how I was feeling and words of encouragement filled my ears. She obviously cared about my health and how I was feeling, and reassured me the side-effects would pass.

Once back at home, I began noticing more of the dreaded side-effects taking place. The ends of my fingers on my left hand began tingling and the skin on both my palms began to feel very dry. Despite taking a range of anti-sickness tablets, my nausea increased. The hiccups from hell returned around 19:00 and continued for almost four hours! Eventually I slept, but woke during the early hours. The feelings of hunger, along with the nausea, continued unabated and I suffered from painful indigestion.

It was now Friday, three days since my second cycle, and my feelings of sickness seemed to know no bounds. I continued taking as many anti-sickness tablets as I was allowed, in the hope they would take away the feelings. I now felt exhausted and began to suffer from feelings of dizziness. The dizziness came without warning, sometimes lasting minutes and sometimes hours. However, that night I managed to sleep well, with only a few interruptions. I woke at 08:00 on Saturday morning and, miracle upon miracle, I didn't feel sick! I noticed that the tingling in my fingers, along with the pain in my jaw when eating or drinking, had ceased. I felt exhausted, but the only real side-effects I was suffering were the fatigue and the dizzy spells.

Monday, I had my bloods taken and my PICC line flushed,

as per normal.

Tuesday arrived and, along with it, my two-weekly meeting with Dr Patel. I told him how I was feeling and concern was written all over his face. He immediately told me to stop taking one of the anti-sickness tablets he had prescribed and then explained that he would withdraw the oxaliplatin from my regime. He was under the impression that this chemical, combined with the anti-sickness tablet, was causing my dizziness and that the oxaliplatin was the cause of my nausea. He would cease the oxaliplatin until my seventh cycle and then reintroduce it at only fifty per cent of the amount I had previously been given.

He reassured me that although ideally oxaliplatin should remain part of my treatment, its effects on curing my cancer were minimal and the other two drugs in my regime, namely folinic acid and fluorouracil, were the main cures. He had kept his word. My quality of life was as important as my treatment and the hope was that withdrawing this chemical would improve my quality of life, without affecting too much the quality of the treatment I was receiving.

Dr Patel had given me knew hope. I left our meeting somewhat happier than when I had arrived. The brakes on my emotional rollercoaster had been pressed just that touch firmer.

Dr Patel had made an appointment for me to visit the hospital the next day, to have an oral review of the medication I was taking. So, on 20th July, I attended as asked. I had a further PICC line flush and met with the pharmacist who told me she had met with Dr Patel earlier that day. Between them, it had been decided I should stop taking my present anti-sickness tablets and take a different one. This tablet was to be placed between my top lip and top gum and left there to dissolve, thus entering my system. I took the tablet as instructed. Guess what? I felt sicker than ever and continued feeling dizzy!

I telephoned the hospital and spoke with Katherine who immediately asked me to attend. Whilst there, I spoke with the duty doctor. Immediately, he stopped the new tablet and put me back on the original ones.

The day continued as it began. I felt nauseous and dizzy, but by the evening the dizziness had ceased. The feelings of sickness continued for two further days until I felt 'normal.' It was now only two days before my dreaded third cycle, so I would only have two nausea-free days before it all began again!

It had been a game of trial and error in recent times. The 'error' was not the fault of any medical staff in any way. The 'error' was me. It was my body which was reacting adversely to the medication. The medical staff tried different things to reduce my reactions. I was feeling pretty low at this time. I was dreading my next cycle and the days that would follow: the nausea, the pains, the sleeplessness and fatigue that would accompany me. My emotional rollercoaster was travelling quicker than ever, in the wrong direction, and my views on a particular issue changed during these days. I had always held the view that any treatment that could prolong a patient's life should be carried out. I had seen chemotherapy patients on the television and heard their words on the radio, denying themselves the treatment which would prolong them living. I could not comprehend the mentality of not undergoing treatment which would allow them to live longer, even if that treatment would only buy them a short time. My view had been that if I was in their position, I would surely want the treatment that would give me those few extra months of life, allowing me to experience precious times with my loved ones, doing special things with them for as long as possible.

Again I had been ignorant. Now I knew exactly why they would deny themselves their treatment. I now knew exactly why they would refuse their 'medicine,' a decision that would, undoubtedly, reduce their life expectancy. My view had flipped one hundred and eighty degrees. Now I would always know why someone would refuse their treatment. It was their decision, their body, their life and no one else's. If they chose not to succumb to the terrible side-effects which would inevitably follow their cycles, it was their choice. Having experienced only 'minor' side-effects compared to others, I would never question their decisions again, ever.

On Monday 25th July, I attended the hospital for another flushing and to have my bloods taken. By now I was becoming accustomed to these visits. Blood was taken, via my line, and the red liquid easily filled the small test tubes. This blood was then taken to another department and analysed to check, amongst other things, the levels of my red and white blood cells. Any problems and I would receive a telephone call. So far, I had received no telephone calls regarding these levels.

Tuesday, all too quickly, followed Monday and I attended the hospital. My third cycle was soon underway. This was going to be different. I would have no oxaliplatin pumped into me. I had no idea whether this would change the way I would feel in the coming days. My experience so far was that, following chemotherapy, I felt sick, had painful hiccups that lasted for hours, pains in my jaw, pains in my fingertips and a metallic taste in my mouth. My trust was placed wholly in Dr Patel and his staff and I trusted them implicitly. Time would tell. There were no guarantees that removing this drug from my system would make me feel less ill but naturally I went along with it. If the outcome was that I would suffer less severe side-effects, I was willing to try it. Who wouldn't? The doctor and nurses were helping me and I felt in very safe hands. At the back of my mind, I had the thought that the removal of this drug may be detrimental to the ultimate goal of removing Mr C from me completely. It was a natural worry for me. The reason I was having this treatment was to 'clean' my system, to kill any cancer still lingering within me and I certainly didn't want to have to undergo further treatment once my regime was completed. My future happiness was in the hands of the good doctor. So far, he hadn't failed me and had always been honest and caring. If the removal of the oxaliplatin helped how I was feeling physically and the other two chemicals completed their task, then all well and good. After all, by this stage I'd only had two cycles and they had made me feel almost constantly sick, so God only knew what I'd feel like after twelve!

Louise and Fiona prepared my pump for fitting and we spoke about my upcoming holiday. In three days, my wife and I, along with our son and the family dog, would travel from the south of England to the North, for a week's holiday on the shores of Lake Windermere in the beautiful English Lake District. There we would join my wife's father, her sister and family and their dog for a welcome break from all the madness. I hoped with all my heart that I would be able to enjoy our time together and not be feeling sick and suffering the side-effects which had accompanied me following each cycle so far.

That evening something peculiar occurred, or rather didn't. When I ate I felt no pain. The 'mother of all hiccups' did not visit and, upon handling anything cold, nothing happened. My temperature was normal and I felt good. Yes, I awoke early the following morning, starving as usual and, yes, I felt weak, but other than felling fatigued and looking pale, it was the best I'd felt since my treatment began. With renewed hope, I watched the hours tick by, waiting to see if my nausea returned. It didn't. Day became evening and I continued taking my medication, cleaning my teeth and checking my temperature and waiting. That night I slept well. I was now used to sleeping with my pump attached, safely housed in my bum bag, and had mastered the technique of spending the vast majority of my sleeping hours prone on my back. Obviously, I woke early, feeling hungry, but that was it.

Night became day, which passed, and soon it was Thursday. I travelled to the hospital and still felt well. Upon my arrival, Louise immediately noticed a change in me. She remarked that I looked much better than she had seen me looking for weeks. I told her I felt good and she could clearly see the relief and joy in my face. We hugged each other and my eyes filled with tears. Again, these were not tears of sadness, but tears of joy, hope and relief.

Suddenly, with the removal of that one chemical, my life had changed. It was as though some medieval torturer had ceased his work, freed me from my shackles and allowed me to go about my daily business almost as normal. I was not suffering any dizziness and was not feeling sick. To me, it was as though a miracle had occurred, the miracle of not having oxaliplatin flowing through me. The good doctor and those working with him were now applying the brakes to my rollercoaster.

With my pump removed, Louise and Katherine both wished me a good holiday. Both reassured me, as they had always done, telling me not to worry and to have a relaxing week. They told me to 'listen to my body' and when it told me to rest, I should do so. The week was to be a time to try and forget what had gone on previously. There would be the inevitable chats about how I was feeling and what I was going through, but it was a week of no arranged hospital visits. Should I need to visit the nearest hospital whilst I was away, that wouldn't be a problem. Katherine would make the necessary arrangements and I would be looked after. She reminded me that take away food was 'not an option' and I smiled, and this time I reassured her!

As I drove away from the hospital, along the narrow, meandering driveway, I saw something from the corner of my eye. It was the resident peacock. Peculiarly he, or she, was facing me and I was around twenty metres away. A split second later, the peacock was gone, scuttling out of sight into the undergrowth. In that moment I knew somehow that my week away would pass without incident.

Arriving home, my wife and I finished packing. I say 'we' finished packing but that is being generous. I finished packing my case and she finished hers, my son's and packed all the pet things which were needed!

I still felt well, no pains, no hiccups, no sickness and no temperature spikes. I was now a quarter of the way through my FOLFOX regime, which had now become the FOLF regime, as the oxaliplatin had been removed, although only temporarily. It seemed that the removal of this chemical had taken away almost all of my side-effects. This was a huge relief; however, I was unable to lose the feeling that, although removing the oxaliplatin massively reduced my side-effects, this may have a detrimental effect on the main reason I was undergoing treatment, to rid my body of any possible cancer. Again, a new 'trial and error' phase had entered my life. By not having oxaliplatin running through my veins, my quality of life had clearly increased, but would this affect the whole reason for this treatment? Time would tell. Had I been told that the removal of one third of my treatment added a large risk to my cancer not being destroyed, I would have continued with the full treatment. That was not what I was being told. I was being told that the removal of this part of the treatment would have a minimal adverse effect on my body being rid of cancer and that risk, to me, was worth the rewards.

I had complete faith in the oncologist guiding my treatment and I followed his lead. After all, my experience with cancer had been a very short one and he had many years of experience in his specialized field. Who was I to even question his judgement? I always felt supremely confident that, under Dr Patel's expert guidance, I would finish my treatment and my cancer would be destroyed completely. If he thought that by removing one of the fluids being pumped into me my chances of winning this battle were not significantly reduced, that was absolutely fine by me. To not suffer the side-effects I had become accustomed to and to have the risk of me being cancer-free, reduced by only one or two percentage points, was no problem to me. The medical staff who had looked after me, so far, had not failed me. They had my complete trust and had always been correct. I trusted Dr Patel implicitly. My life was, literally, in his hands and I had no doubt he would perform his work to the absolute best of his ability. He was there to guide me, treat me and, ultimately, cure me, and I would take his advice without question. He hadn't failed me yet and I was confident it would be that way in the future.

CHAPTER ELEVEN

Prison

It was now 29th July 2016, the first day of our holiday. My wife and I had discussed our journey. It would take us from the south coast of England, through the Midlands, past Birmingham, then past Manchester and onward, towards Scotland. It was a journey of some three hundred miles, taking around five to six hours, travelling by car. I would drive; however, should I feel fatigued at any point, my wife would take over.

We loaded the car with cases, supplies for the journey, dog beds, dog food and off we all went. I felt fine, not ill, in no pain and had high hopes. The change of scenery would, surely, take my mind off things that had passed and were yet to pass. The journey passed without incident, with our dog sleeping most of the way and our son spending the majority of the journey wearing headphones.

We arrived at our destination safely some six hours later. I managed to drive the whole way although by the time the journey was over, I felt extremely tired. We unloaded the luggage into the log cabin which was to be our home for the next week. The cabin was situated on the shores of the lake with a beautiful view of the breath-taking scenery. We were greeted by my wife's sister, her family and their pooch, who went by the name of Murphy. Our Bassett and Murphy got along famously, playing and chasing each other, until one succumbed to exhaustion. One hundred per cent of the time, it was the Bassett!

Our days were ones of laughter, sightseeing and relaxation. My sister-in-law, her family, Murphy and our son would go walking nearby, admiring the scenery, and ascending and descending the nearby pikes. I was unable to join them on most of these trips as I just didn't have the energy to do so. I wanted, so much, to walk with them, deep into the forests which surrounded the lake but physically I was unable to. I was beginning to suffer from a higher level of fatigue than I had done and was forced to listen to my body. My wife and I would take a sedentary boat trip or just wander the shores of the lake, staying close to the cabin. Evenings would see the families joining each other in either of the cabins. The alcohol would flow, the music would play and good food would be eaten. On most occasions, I would have to cut short our meetings as my tiredness overcame me, forcing an early retirement from the merriment. All concerned knew what treatment I was having and understood why I had to leave them enjoying the long nights.

Thankfully, I had no need to contact Katherine and no need to visit Lancaster Infirmary. The days and evenings passed all too quickly, without any real concerns.

Towards the end of our holiday, we decided to eat our evening meal at a local restaurant. As we readied ourselves for our evening out, something caught my eye. I was cleaning my teeth and glancing in the mirror. A deep red mark, about the size of a human thumbnail, took my concentration. It was positioned just above my top lip, on the left side, about halfway between the bottom of my nose and the left corner of my mouth. There was no sensation accompanying it, no pain, no itchiness and it just seemed to appear. It wasn't there one minute and the next it was. It looked as though I had been bitten by an insect, but I was sure I hadn't. There was no central raising of the skin; in fact, there was no texture or feeling to it whatsoever. It didn't increase or decrease in size or colour, it just was! Was this the start of something I'd only ever heard of fleetingly, something referred to as 'chemo tan'? I had heard stories of people suffering from patches of red skin following chemotherapy, but had not, up until now, experienced it.

As I continued getting ready, I kept my eye on my upper lip. There was no change. The mark showed no increase in size or colour. I spoke to my wife and told her that I now didn't now want to go out with my red mark accompanying me. I was very conscious of it and I had visions of people staring at 'my little red friend'. I immediately wanted to cancel the evening for myself. I needn't have worried or become so vain. My wife had a very simple solution. Foundation! She applied the makeup expertly to my top lip and the red spot began to slowly disappear. The colour blended well and the mark became invisible within seconds. Furthermore, it was almost impossible for anyone to detect that there was a thin disguise covering my top lip: I was clean-shaven, so there was no five o'clock shadow on the rest of my face to cover.

Foundation applied, my evening was able to continue. No one noticed my foundation application or at least no one commented. I do not know to this day whether anyone noticed but that simple solution allowed my evening to continue without worry. Again, an answer was found to a problem, albeit very small.

The next day came and my little red friend had gone back to where he came. He was no longer. The holiday drew to a close and I had no further issues. Yes, I awoke early each day and I felt tired, but I had successfully accomplished the week away. It was time that was needed, a chance to relax with loved ones. They knew what I was going through, always offering their heartfelt support, never questioning or judging and always offering their love.

It was now time to get back to reality and during our journey home my thoughts turned to my upcoming cycle. It was just a few days until my fourth treatment would begin. After this cycle, I would be a third of the way through my regime. My spirits were lifted immeasurably by my recent lack of side-effects and I was now not dreading my next treatment. The removal of the oxaliplatin seemed to have been successful in minimising these effects. I had no dizziness, sickness or any of the other ailments I had succumbed to and just felt tired for the majority of the time. I guessed this was the cumulative effects of the treatment and was something I could deal with. It was, undoubtedly, the happiest time I'd experienced since my regime began.

Following more taking of blood, my fourth treatment came and went. Steroids, antihistamines and anti-sickness liquids were pumped into me, followed by folinic acid and fluorouracil. My pump was attached and off I went. I suffered no hiccups, no dizziness and only felt a very mild sense of nausea, which lasted two days. Although I was still being cautious when handling cold items, I had no pains in my fingertips. The pump emptied its contents into my system and was then removed. I was still taking my medicines and still waking during the early hours, feeling hungry. Other than this, my main concern was fatigue. Following the removal of my pump, I went to bed; that was Thursday 11th August and I remained in bed, almost constantly, until the following Monday. Other than waking during the early hours and eating before returning to bed, this was the pattern which would, unbeknown to me then, continue throughout my remaining treatment.

I had now completed four of my twelve cycles and to go with my ever-increasing fatigue I began to notice some further physical changes occurring. My hair to the front of my head began thinning. It was a subtle change, but a clear one. The hair on my arms, legs, chest, stomach and underarms began to disappear and my eyelashes below my eyes seemed to shrink in length and reduce in amount. Strangely, the hair around my genitals remained. Why was this the case? No one seemed to know. My two-weekly visit to Dr Patel threw no light on the matter. He reassured me that any lost hair would return following the conclusion of my treatment but was unable to answer why I lost the hair on my body but with the exception of the hair around my genitals, which remained. He seemed unmoved by my werewolf tendencies in reverse!

During this meeting, Dr Patel informed me of something that he was uncomfortable with, namely my platelet count. He pointed out that my platelet level had fallen to eighty-eight when the number should have been nearer to one hundred and fifty. This was of concern because should I cut myself, or suffer injury, my blood would not coagulate properly and I was at risk of losing a large amount of blood. It was something he would be keeping a very close eye on. Of course, this was concerning, not only to the good doctor but also to me. I became more careful than ever when going about my daily business. I did not want to cut myself in any way. Even the smallest cut, which most people would just cover with a plaster and forget about, could cause me an issue, undoubtedly resulting in an unplanned visit to the hospital. I had enough planned visits to the hospital, thank you very much!

The following Monday, 22nd August, my bloods were taken and my PICC line flushed. I had now become so accustomed to my bloods being taken that it became part of my 'being.' Louise performed these tasks with the utmost skills and the following day my fifth treatment was completed. Again, I had no oxaliplatin pumped into me and with pump attached I left, my little red book in my hand. Again, I experienced the early morning wake-up calls and fatigue, but not much else. Two days later, the pump was empty and was removed. When I got home, I went to bed where I mostly remained until Monday.

As the Monday was a summer bank holiday, my PICC line was flushed and my bloods taken on the Tuesday and, later that day, a further meeting with Dr Patel took place. He assured me that I was doing well and explained that the fatigue I was suffering from was perfectly normal for someone undergoing treatment and that it was the cumulative effect of that treatment causing my tiredness. He told me I should be drinking three litres of water per day to help clean my liver and system of any chemicals which had been pumped into me. Three litres! This was something I found difficult to do and managed one to two litres at best. I told him I was not sunbathing or gardening, and I was cleaning my teeth regularly. I asked him if I was allowed to drink alcohol. He replied that for each pint of beer or lager I drank, I should drink three pints of water. Water, water everywhere, I thought to myself.

Dr Patel made me happy, almost joyous, when he told me that he was not going to introduce any oxaliplatin to my next cycle. However, he reminded me that cycle seven would include the dreaded chemical, but only at fifty per cent of the level I had had during my first two treatments. Dr Patel had now applied more pressure to the brakes on my emotional rollercoaster.

During the periods between my cycles, I would receive visits from various friends and colleagues. These would normally occur during the working week, around lunchtime. I would be making myself comfortable, assuming my normal resting position on my couch and nodding off, when there would be a tap on the window. I would open my eyes to see the smiling faces of either my brother-in-law, Matthew, or my good friend Patrick, peering at me before they were invited in for a coffee and catch-up.

I was visited by other work friends and by a good friend whom I will call Andrew. Andrew was a fireman and would tell me of what 'shouts' he had been to. He also supplied me with various DVDs to watch to break up the long days. These visits were always welcomed and cheered me up no end. They all visited regularly and no matter how I was feeling, I always felt better for seeing them. They became my eyes on the outside world as my own world had been consumed by what I was going through, taking a back seat whilst I was having treatment.

My mother contacted me daily by telephone. Because of their ages, travelling to see me was difficult for my parents. Both were in their eighties and neither one of them now drove. I visited them when I was able, but it wasn't as often as we all would have liked. Whist I was having chemotherapy, my mother telephoned me each evening without fail. She always enquired how I was feeling and how I was coping. Even when I was at my lowest ebb, I would reassure her that I was doing well. I always wanted to protect my parents as best I could from what Mr C was doing to me and always told them I was doing well, even if that wasn't always necessarily the case. My mother's calls always lifted my spirits, each and every time.

Several attitudes of mine changed during these long months of chemotherapy. I began to see a number of things differently. For instance, if I was driving my car along a road and another driver performed some questionable manoeuvre, such as pulling out of a side road in front of me, causing me to brake, or overtaking me and pulling in sharply in front of me, causing me once again to brake, it didn't really matter. Prior to my diagnosis I would have probably flashed my headlights in their direction or cussed at them loudly. Now, those little indiscretions didn't matter. I would just let it pass with no negativity towards the other driver. It meant nothing and I didn't view it as a problem which, we all know ninety-nine times out of a hundred, it really isn't. No damage had been done and very little time had been added to my journey by their driving. My attitude now was 'so what?' Little actions that had previously tested my patience really did not affect me anymore. Being diagnosed with a life-threatening illness tends to focus your mind. The small things that may have annoyed you during your everyday life now just evaporated into thin air. They didn't matter anymore and shouldn't have before. They just weren't worth worrying about now.

A further change occurred during my chemotherapy period. Prior to diagnosis, my daughter and her partner's relationship came to an end. It was no surprise to either me or my wife as they were both young and things had moved very quickly. They had set up a home together and our granddaughter was the fruit of their relationship. Soon after she was born, the relationship faltered and their relationship ended. This was not unusual in any way but following the breakup, my granddaughter's father, a young man called Dave, went off the rails, big style. He began drinking, consuming vast quantities of alcohol at each sitting. It was his way of coping with the ending of their relationship. People cope with bad experiences in different ways and this was his way.

Now, when I've had a drink, I will chat a little and become mellow. Some like to sing, some like to dance, some like to talk and some like to fight. Dave liked to fight. In fact, he didn't want to just fight he wanted to take on the world! Whilst everything was stable in his world, there were no problems but when life became difficult and unstable, he drank. Drinking changed his personality completely and he had no cares. He would do what he wanted to, whether it was legal or not, and would end up fighting once the alcohol flowed into him. He controlled these emotions by avoiding drink, but once his world had changed for the worse, he sought solace through alcohol. He knew it was a dangerous path to follow, but it seemed the only way he knew, the only way he could cope with his demons. Trouble swiftly followed. After a number of these drinking sessions and the trouble that accompanied them, he ended up being sentenced to four years imprisonment.

I had wanted nothing more to do with Dave. He had left his daughter, left my granddaughter almost fatherless, and I was unsure I could forgive him. He had let himself down, his loved ones down but most of all he had let his daughter down.

During my treatment, my attitude changed. I found out where he was serving his time and wrote to him. Letters were exchanged and my wife and I decided we should visit him, taking his daughter with us. He loved the idea and supplied us with a visiting order and arrangements were made. One Saturday morning, we set off on the four-hour journey for our first-ever prison visit. This being our first visit, we literally did not know what to expect. On a Saturday, visiting hours were between 13:45 and 15:45 and we were asked to arrive approximately one hour before visiting began, which we did.

Parking in the visitors' car park, we walked to a small, brick building outside the prison fences which surrounded the prison. The building was entitled Visitors Centre and we entered with trepidation. Inside was a small office where we handed in our identification and visiting order to a prison warden. We were then given a ticket with a number on it. This was our visitor number which was twenty-two, meaning we would be the twenty-second group allowed into the visiting room.

We sat down with the other visitors in the small building and waited. The room was scruffy, dirty and in need of decoration. As time passed, each chair became occupied with people waiting to see their loved ones. We placed our belongings into a small locker as we had been told we were not permitted to take any personal items whatsoever into the prison, with the exception of a small amount of money in coins, so that items could be purchased from the vending machines within the hall. There was also a small café within the hall which sold hot bacon or sausage sandwiches and hot drinks, which the visitors were allowed to purchase for themselves or for those they were visiting.

My granddaughter was around two years old and she joined a number of small children playing with the toys in the small play area. There were a few people around my age within the room waiting but the vast majority of visitors appeared to be in their mid-twenties. Young mothers sat with babies in their arms, toddlers ran around like they owned the place and small children played noisily with toys which had clearly seen better days!

We waited patiently, listening to the chatter which filled the room. Judging by the number of accents being spoken, we weren't the only ones who'd travelled a considerably distance to visit.

At around 13:30, a male prison warden entered the building through the main double doors.

'Numbers 1 to 5, please,' he called out and a number of people rose from their seats and, when all were ready, they followed the warden out of the room towards the main prison. We continued waiting and some ten minutes later the warden returned.

'Numbers 6 to 11, please.'

Those holding those numbers stood and followed the man from the room. The pattern continued and eventually, after what seemed hours but was actually around forty-five minutes, our number was called. A number of people stood, and my wife and I, along with our granddaughter, joined them, and we were led from the room. We all walked along a short path, which led from the visitor centre to the prison, through a metal gate and then through a large, glass-panelled, double door and into the prison. We were all led to a barred door which was opened electronically and finally we walked into a small area which was surrounded by vertical steel bars with similar bars on the roof. Once everyone was standing in this area, the steel barred door behind us closed and a second later the one in front of us slid from left to right. We then exited the barred 'room' following which we were asked to form a single file. A warden then ran a handheld metal detector over each individual and a 'pat down' search followed, with female visitors being attended to by female wardens and male visitors being attended to by male wardens. A handler with a sniffer dog walked around each of us, the dog wagging its tail gleefully as it walked around each of those being searched.

My turn came to be searched. I stood with my arms outstretched to each side and my legs slightly apart. The metal detector was passed slowly over my body only inches from my skin. Having passed the metal detection, my 'pat down' commenced. I had nothing to worry about. I had no illegal substances or items about my person and assumed I would sail through any searches. Unfortunately, I was wrong. The search revealed something under my right sleeve. Immediately, I was asked to roll up my sleeve and I obliged. Hastily, I rolled up my sleeve, revealing the Tubigrip which covered my PICC line.

'What's that?' questioned the burly male, who was in his late twenties.

'That's covering my PICC as I'm undergoing cancer treatment and that is where the chemotherapy enters my body,' I replied.

Those words were enough. The warden said no more and just nodded his head, understandingly. I pulled my sleeve to its original position and I stood, somewhat sheepishly, to one side as the remainder of the group were searched.

I thought to myself about what had just happened. The warden heard the words I said and that had been enough. He didn't want to check under the covering to see if I was being truthful. I had the feeling the words 'cancer' and 'chemotherapy' had been enough to stop his enquiries; either that or it was just my trusting face. Clearly, he was a good judge of character!

Searches completed, one of the wardens opened a wooden door and went inside. Seconds later, he emerged carrying a supply of nappies and baby bottles, filled with powdered baby milk. The nappies and bottles were handed to the young mothers who were carrying their babies. A large double, wooden door was then opened ahead of us and I caught my first view of a prison visitors hall. It was a large area with numerous small round tables spread around the room. At each table sat an inmate either chatting to his visitors or waiting to welcome those visiting him.

As I entered the room, my eyes darted from left to right, then left and right again, as I scoured the room for a sign of Dave. There he was, sat alone at his table, wearing his regulation pair of jeans and short-sleeved shirt. As he saw his daughter for the first time in a long time, his expression changed. He smiled broadly, his white teeth almost shining between his parted lips. His face instantly lit up and he rose to a standing position, so there could be no doubt we would see him. I smiled broadly back at him. I don't think I had ever experienced such delight on a person's face as I did in that instant, the moment Dave first set eyes on his daughter since his incarceration. He held her tight and we all hugged him, as we were permitted to do, before we sat at his table.

His daughter soon became bored and wandered over to the rather sad-looking children's play area in one of the corners of the room, where she played with several children of a similar age.

I bought Dave several cups of coffee and bacon rolls and we chatted about nothing in particular, apart from his daughter. He explained that he was taking a painting and decorating course, courtesy of the prison, and on his release it would be his chosen profession. He had visions of starting a small company when he got out, maybe employing another person. I knew that day was a long way away but I could see the ambition and excitement in his eyes.

Dave told us that he was undertaking further courses such as an alcohol and drug abuse course and he seemed upbeat about his future. He was using the prison gymnasium regularly and doing whatever he could to pass the time whilst he had lost his liberty.

He told us he had his own single cell which was small and that during the day the door was unlocked, meaning he was able to wander around the wing as he pleased. As long as he was in his cell by the time it was lockdown, that being 17:00, there were no issues. He explained that the main problem he faced was a simple one: boredom. The courses he was on and the gym visits didn't fill his day, and passing the remaining time was problematic. He accepted he had done wrong and the resulting loss of his freedom. He clearly regretted the actions which had led him to where he now was and he certainly wasn't one of those individuals who thought he didn't deserve the sentence he had been given; in fact, quite the opposite. He said he deserved his incarceration, he would serve his time and he hoped to rebuild his life. We all knew it would be a long and difficult path for him but worth it in the end. Naturally, my wife and I wished him well and hoped this would be the last time he would be within the walls of one of Her Majesty's hotels but that would be up to only one person – Dave.

As I looked around the large room, something struck me – the age of the vast majority of those housed behind the prison walls. There were very few men in the room above the age of thirty. Out of all the men in there, at least a hundred, you could count the ones over thirty on the fingers of one hand. The rest were in their early- to mid-twenties and, undoubtedly, the vast majority deserved their punishments. They had wronged society and society had its revenge, locking them away for long periods of time. Men in the prime of their lives sat within the walls of this room, surrounded by walls, high fences and countless barred doors and windows, all covered by large numbers of surveillance cameras watching their every move. These young men should have been enjoying their lives, spending time with friends, socialising, building relationships, starting their adult lives but here they were, sitting around tables with their loved ones whom they weren't even allowed to hold in their arms. Should any hugging take place whilst the visits were underway, the wardens dotted around the room would spring into action and stop any 'untoward' behaviour.

It seemed that almost before it had begun our visit was over. We were permitted our parting hugs, with Dave hugging his young daughter tightly, holding her close to him for as long as possible. It was a sad sight to see, but it was what it was. Dave knew it was his fault he was in this position and certainly didn't blame anyone else. My wife and I hugged him and we said our goodbyes.

As I left the room, I looked back in Dave's direction. He was sitting at his table, just watching us leave. I gave him a thumbs up and he returned the gesture and smiled once more. We left the hall and made our way back to the visitors' centre where we collected what we had left in our locker. We left the prison grounds and drove to the hotel we were staying in for the night before our journey home began. Following my first prison visit, I took many thoughts away with me from that place but the overwhelming one was one of great sadness.

Further visits would follow until Dave's release and each time the feelings of sadness were always foremost in my mind. Dave served his time and began rebuilding his life with a new partner and a new baby son. Naturally, my wife and I wish him well and at least we know who to call on when our hallway needs painting!

CHAPTER TWELVE

Bananas!

It was now 5th September 2016, the day before my sixth cycle. I had begun working and had done so for several weeks. Although I say working, it was only on a limited basis. I would work part time during the weeks between my cycles, leaving for any hospital visits I needed to attend. I worked mainly in the mornings, doing three or four hours, before I became tired and needed to rest. I would just let my boss know and, thankfully, it wasn't a problem.

So, I attended my appointment. Blood was taken and my line was flushed and away I went, before returning the next day for number six. However, there was a problem. My platelet count had dropped even further than before, down to a count of eighty-four. It was simple: as my count had fallen again and was so low, my treatment could not go ahead. It would be too dangerous for me to undergo any further treatment until the count rose and my next round of chemotherapy was postponed for a week in the hope that my count would rise sufficiently. It was not what I would call a devastating blow but it was a blow. Everything had been running smoothly up until now. With the withdrawal of the dreaded oxaliplatin, I had not suffered the terrible side-effects. Yes, the hair had almost disappeared completely from my limbs, chest and stomach and the hair above my forehead was definitely thinning, along with my lower eyelashes, but these were things I could easily cope with. I continued waking at 'stupid o'clock' and was still suffering the hunger pangs and the fatigue but really that was about it. Now, thanks to a low count, my treatment would be extended for at least a week. My last treatment was due on 29th November 2016, but now it would run into December. I had visions of my treatment having to continue into the Christmas period, an important time for many families, including mine.

My seventh cycle would see the reintroduction of the oxaliplatin, albeit at fifty per cent strength and, once more, I envisaged the side-effects this chemical would produce. I desperately wanted to be well over Christmas and now that was in doubt. Again, the wheels on my rollercoaster seemed to be speeding up again when recently they had been slowing. I feared what Christmas would bring but there would be little I could do about it.

I was told to rest over the next week and advised to do as little as possible. Of course, I would do as I was advised. As I began to leave the oncology department, the lovely Louise hugged me. She could see how deflated I was by the recent news I had received. As she hugged me, she whispered into my right ear.

'Eat some bananas, my cherub, it may help.'

Over the next few days, I rested and took Louise's advice. Now, bananas are not necessarily my favourite fruit and I did not consume excessive amounts of them but I did eat one a day, in the hope they may help. I rested even more than usual, didn't attend work or really even leave the house. I desperately wanted my cycles to begin again because the sooner they continued, the sooner they finished and any lingering cancer cells would be gone. The days dragged by, hour by hour, but eventually, pass they did and it was time for another visit to see Louise and have my line flushed and my bloods taken, yet again.

The day after my bloods were taken, I attended the hospital and learnt that, amazingly, my platelet count had risen to one hundred and twenty-eight! This was the highest it had been since my cycles had begun. My platelet count had been steadily falling since my first cycle, but had now shot up. I caught Louise's eye, winked at her and she winked back and my sixth cycle began. As Louise attached my line to the mobile drip stand, she explained her banana rationale to me. There was no scientific proof that the bananas would help but she had known a number of patients who had been in a similar position to mine where this fruit had actually seemed to help. Since that day, I try to eat one banana a day. In the saying, 'an apple a day keeps the doctor away,' I have substituted the word 'apple' with the word 'banana'!

The following week passed without any dramas. A little constipation, early morning awakenings and pangs of hunger and, following my pump removal, fatigue. The usual few days spent mainly in bed followed and then a PICC line flush and it was time to see Dr Patel once more. This visit to the good doctor threw up another curve ball. My white blood count was now beginning to fall! So, having managed to control my platelet count, I was now faced with something more sinister. Dr Patel explained that the white blood cells were extremely important as they were part of the body's immune system, helping the body to fight infections and diseases. Fan-bloody-tastic, I thought to myself. Dr Patel told me that I would be required to begin a course of self-administered injections, starting five days after chemotherapy. The reason the white blood cell count had fallen was due to the cumulative effects of my treatment. This was a common occurrence and would, hopefully, be rectified by the injections. I would have to inject myself in my stomach once a day for three days after each of my cycles, to boost my white blood cell count. This would improve my immune system and hopefully allow my body to fight any infection which may occur. I would need the injections until this blood count rose to an acceptable level. He further explained that my next cycle, number seven, would include oxaliplatin at fifty per cent of what I had originally been prescribed. The very word oxaliplatin sent shivers down my spine.

The day came for another taking of bloods and PICC flush, followed by my seventh cycle. It was around 08:00 on the day of my next cycle when my telephone rang. It was Fiona from the hospital. She asked me to attend the hospital immediately as the results of my latest blood analysis were worrying them. The counts had dropped once more.

I went straight to the hospital and a further two test tubes of blood were taken and the results swiftly returned. My platelet count had fallen to one hundred and my white blood cell count had fallen even further. My seventh cycle was now in serious doubt. Phone calls were made between Katherine and the doctors and, after much deliberation, it was decided that treatment should continue. I was thankful of this decision as any further delays would just push the 'finishing line' further away. I wanted the treatment completed and as soon as possible. The longer it dragged on, the worse it was.

I was now beginning to see some light at the end of the tunnel, a tunnel that seemed to be going on forever. The end was in sight and, when it was reached, my journey could end. Anything that lengthened that journey, in turn accelerated the wheels on my emotional rollercoaster, sending it in the wrong direction.

So, steroids, antihistamines and anti-sickness medicine flowed into my body, followed by the folinic acid, the fluorouracil and the dreaded oxaliplatin. My pump was attached and the appropriate tablets supplied, along with three syringes filled with a transparent liquid which I was to begin self-administering in five days. I would inject the liquid directly into my stomach area and, all being well, it would serve its purpose.

I left the hospital wary that the dreaded 'O' was flowing through my system once again. I hoped beyond hope that, as it was only half the dose I had received before, my side-effects would remain minimal. The days passed and my side-effects continued as they had been during the weeks following the removal of the dreaded 'O'. They remained 'minimal' despite this chemical now travelling through my body. My pump was removed and constipation followed although that was now easily controlled. Fatigue set in but, other than that, I felt fine. No sickness, no dizziness, no pains in my jaw or fingertips and no hiccups occurred. I injected myself as I had been instructed and disposed each empty syringe into the sharps box I had been supplied with.

My cycles continued along with blood tests, line flushes and visits to the good doctor. The same side-effects that followed my third cycle continued, although the hair on my body was no longer visible other than on my head, my face and around my genitals. My lower eyelashes remained although somewhat shorter in length and number than ever before and were difficult to see. My taste buds were not functioning as they should and I was unable to taste the strong flavours in foods. I could have had the hottest curry known and probably not even raised a sweat. The cumulative effects of the treatment were clearly taking their toll.

The injections continued, along with the oral medication and cycles nine and ten passed. Following my tenth treatment, the good doctor stopped prescribing the injections as they had successfully aided my white blood cell count and were no longer required.

Cycle eleven was now only a day away, when I noticed something odd with my PICC line. The part of the line which was protruding from my inner elbow and held in place to the surface by its 'fixing' had altered. Somehow the protruding line seemed longer than I had previously noticed it to be.

I attended the hospital to have my PICC line flushed and my bloods taken and told Fiona my concerns regarding my line. Katherine was immediately called and the length of the protruding part of my line was measured, using a good old-fashioned twelve-inch ruler. Following the measurements, concern was etched on both Katherine's and Fiona's faces. According to the measurements, my line had moved two inches and the visible part of my line was now two inches longer! Obviously, this was bad news. It meant that if my eleventh treatment was given, it could cause significant damage to my body. Katherine explained that with the line having moved these two inches, the internal end of the line, which was supposed to be next to my heart, now wasn't. If the acid which was in the chemicals being pumped into me came into contact with my bodily tissues, without being rapidly pumped away, it could burn that tissue away and it was possible that it would never grow back. It could cause me great pain and, possibly, cause any number of complications.

I was now scared again, more scared than I had been since I learnt I would have to undergo chemotherapy. The wheels on my rollercoaster, which had been slowed considerably over the last few weeks, began gathering momentum.

Immediately an X-ray was arranged and within twenty minutes or so this was duly performed. The results were passed to Dr Patel and Dr Cosford, the latter being the gentleman who originally inserted my line. After a wait of what seemed hours but was actually only around twenty minutes, a decision was made. Chemotherapy would continue. If the line moved anymore at all, it would need removing and a new one would need to be inserted, no question.

I was relieved beyond words. I had come so far on this journey having had ten of my twelve scheduled cycles and the end of treatment was in sight. All I wanted was to undergo the remaining two cycles with no more hiccups and continue my life, as it had been previously. The rollercoaster began slowing once again.

On 22nd November 2016, my penultimate chemotherapy treatment began. It was the same as it had been over the past months. I was now experienced in the pattern of my regime. My body was becoming more fatigued with each cycle and I spent more time than ever sleeping. It was as though my body was telling me, 'No more – I've had enough now,' but now I was almost there. I had just one cycle left and it couldn't come quickly enough. I became excited. Just one more and then I could enjoy Christmas with my loved ones and, enjoy it I fucking well would! My wife, son, daughter, granddaughter, mother, father and all my loved ones could enjoy it with me. Christmas would be extra special this year, the most wonderful since my childhood. There was just one more hurdle to accomplish, just one more round of chemotherapy to endure, one more pump attachment, one pump removal and one more bout of side-effects to suffer.

On 28th November 2016, my bloods were taken, my line was flushed and another X-ray taken, to ensure my line hadn't moved any further. It hadn't.

The following day, another appointment with Dr Patel confirmed all was well for me to have my twelfth and final cycle, scheduled for the 6th December.

My wife, who had accompanied me to all my meetings with the oncologist, asked him a question regarding my treatment and we were both shocked by his answer. She asked him how long the chemicals that had been pumped into me over the last six months would remain within me, floating around in my blood stream. We had both assumed it would be a lengthy period, with the chemicals slowly dissipating inside me, until they were no more. Our estimates were very frugal.

'Although the answer to your question is not exactly known, some have said the chemicals could remain within your system for approximately ten years,' Dr Patel answered.

Both my wife and I nearly fell off our chairs!

'Christ,' I thought to myself. 'I am going to have this shit flowing inside me for the next TEN years!'

A further question cropped up. I had heard of something called 'chemo brain.' This was something that had bothered me for some time and referred to the way the chemicals affected people's minds, causing memory loss amongst other things. The good doctor was unable to confirm whether this was true or not, but did say there was no scientific evidence to support my worries, but he didn't rule it out either. I guess only time will tell.

The next day I visited the hospital once more to check my

line hadn't moved. Further measurements were taken and another X-ay appointment was made for 5th December. The X-ray, along with the taking of bloods and the flushing of my line, took place that day as scheduled and all was well. No further issues occurred and the green light was given for me to have my twelfth and final cycle.

My day arrived – 6th December 2016. I awoke with a sense of excitement. My last cycle was to begin in a matter of hours. Following its completion and the removal of my pump, my PICC line, which had become part of my very existence over the last six months, could be removed. It would signal the completion of chemotherapy for me. The brakes on my rollercoaster were now being applied with maximum force and it was slowing very rapidly. It was now only a short time before it stopped its journey completely and I could unfasten the seatbelt which had constrained me for so long, before exiting for the last time. This particular journey was now almost at an end.

My emotions had now become mixed. I was elated that following my last cycle, no more chemicals would be pumped into me and my side-effects would end. I knew I would feel weak and fatigued for some while yet but, with the passing of each day, I would gain a little in strength and become less tired. My body would begin another journey, the journey back to normality. The hair on my body would return and my sleep pattern would become normal. I wouldn't need to flush the toilet twice after each visit. I could use whichever towels I wished and my laundry could be washed with other people's. I would not need to clean my teeth and gargle with the foul-tasting mouthwash after everything I ate. My darkest days would, surely, be behind me and with each passing day they would become more distant.

I also felt great sadness. My meetings with Katherine, Fiona and Louise, along with the good doctor would cease. I would miss them immensely. The past six months had been traumatic, not only for me but for those I knew and loved, and these people had literally nursed me through it. We had laughed and joked together and they had become a huge part of my life. Without them, I would not be writing this now. Mr C had visited me, entered without permission, trashed the place and, together, we had fought 'Him'. This battle was now coming to an end and it was only a short time until we knew whether or not we had been successful, or we needed to step back, regroup and fight on.

So, my last cycle took place without any problems. Tablets were consumed and no extra side-effects took place. The pump performed magically once more, as each one had, emptying the fluorouracil into my bloodstream, slowly deflating as it did so, until the balloon inside it withered itself down until it resembled a very small, freshly outstretched condom!

I returned to the hospital and entered the oncology department to have my pump removed and my PICC line flushed before its removal. I carried a small zipped-up holdall with me, containing six bottles of wine, several large tins of chocolates and a thank-you card, which I intended to give to

Katherine, Louise and Fiona following the removal of my line. They had all guided me through, undoubtedly, the worst period of my life. They had acted professionally throughout our meetings and their professionalism was only outweighed by the care they showed. They all cared when I felt ill, when I was afraid, when I was nervous, when I was ignorant, when I was emotional, and they cared that by the time my treatment was over, I would be well again. I felt that, although it was a job for these people, that was only a very small part of it. They were there to help and care for their patients, to see them be victorious in their battles and to be able to live their lives once more. They were there for all their patients, without exception and, ultimately, they wanted to make a difference.

Louise removed my pump for the last time and flushed my line before removing the attachment which was holding the visible end of my line in place. She took the access cap from the end of my line, held the line in her hand and pulled. I saw the line rapidly exiting the small hole on the inside of my right elbow until the end which had sat just above my heart for almost six months also exited the hole.

The removal of my line took between one and two seconds and that was it! My regime was completed. I thanked Louise for everything she had done for since we met and I hugged her tightly. I entered Katherine's office carrying the holdall, which I unzipped. I removed the contents and placed them on her desk.

'These are for you, Louise and Fiona for helping me in my hour of need.'

We hugged and Louise and Fiona joined us and I thanked them once more. I hugged the three of them and I left the department, still clutching my little red book in my right hand. I left the hospital, entered my car. My eyes filled with tears as I began the short journey home.

CHAPTER THIRTEEN

Endgame

My journey was, now, almost over. My rollercoaster was grinding to a halt more rapidly than ever before. It had taken me to the top of peaks, only then to descend swiftly to the bottom of numerous troughs. Now, finally, it was travelling up towards the summit of the last peak and I hoped that when it got there, I could get off this ride and never begin the journey again. The last bridge left to cross was a CT scan. Hopefully this would confirm that all the suffering of over a year had been worth it.

My family had endured so much on this journey. My wife had seen me every day of my suffering and had been close by my side every step of the way, always showing her love and support. When I had been short-tempered, she was there; when I was upset, she was there; when I was frightened, she was there; when I was in pain, she was there, always supporting me. My children offered me their love and support throughout. They had seen their father in his darkest of days and their love shone brightly, parting the dark clouds which surrounded me. My family were always there, helping me take the steps that had to be taken. My mother and father saw me, their youngest son, undergo a life-saving operation and chemotherapy, telephoning me each and every night, making sure I was doing OK. My father said to me that he would willingly swap places with me if he could. What left his lips was not just talk, he meant it and I knew he meant it. My best friend, Patrick, had visited regularly, always cheering me with every visit and offering love and support. My brother-in-law Matthew, and my friend Andrew visited, offering love and support and planning good times once I was well. My sister-in-law and her husband spoke to me regularly, always giving me encouragement and support. Sarah, someone I barely knew, heard of my plight, and began messaging me. Her life had been blighted by Mr C from a young age and she knew, to some extent, what I had been suffering, and took the time to support me on my journey. The doctors and nursing staff supported and cared for me. My work colleagues and my boss supported me, with one of them running five kilometres, my name emblazoned on her back! All these people had supported me and I knew I would never forget the support, friendship and love I received.

My greatest fear now was that, despite the love, support and treatment I had received, 'He' was still lurking within me, hiding in some dark corner or orifice, disguising himself, blending in with the surroundings just as a chameleon would do, waiting to appear as if from nowhere and intending to continue wreaking havoc within. My upcoming scan would give me the answers.

On 3rd January 2017, I underwent my scan. By this time I felt absolutely fine, other than still being fatigued. The hair, which had visibly disappeared from my body, was already returning and the hair on my forehead was thickening once more. Thankfully, my hair colour had not changed! I had no problems with my tastebuds, and my sleep pattern was now normal.

In the waiting room, it was just me and my wife. I changed into the hospital gown and drank the barium (which had not improved in taste!) over the hour before my scan, as had been the case before.

The door to the waiting room opened and in walked a female, who appeared slightly older than me. She was followed by a male who was in his mid-twenties. Both sat near to me and my wife. I assumed that the two were related, probably mother and son. A nurse approached them and the male was asked to visit a small cubicle and change into the customary hospital gown. A few minutes later, he emerged, adorned in his gown and took his seat again. I couldn't help but wonder what his ailment was. Perhaps he needed an X-ray on a previously broken bone which had not healed properly, or a scan on some bodily part that was causing some minor issue. After all, he was so young, looked well, just a young man in the prime of his life.

He sat waiting patiently next to the lady who was thumbing through a magazine, just as my wife was doing. No words were exchanged between us, something quite normal for the British when strangers are close by. A nurse approached carrying a drinking container, similar to the one I was drinking from. She placed it on the table directly in front of the young man.

'If you can drink that slowly over the next hour, that would be good,' she said.

I knew exactly what the male had been asked to consume. The young man was quick to reply.

'Does it taste as bad as the last time?' he asked with a smile on his face.

I looked up at the ceiling, thinking to myself, 'Are you taking the piss?' No answer entered my mind.

This man was young and looked so fit and healthy. When I was in my mid-twenties, I was out with friends, meeting new people, enjoying life, as the vast majority of people that age do. Yet this young man was sitting next to me, sipping from a container which contained barium and clearly it wasn't his first experience of drinking the white liquid. He was drinking the fluid which would 'light' up his insides, just as I was, but I was about twice his age, had lived a life, had two grown-up children, a granddaughter, owned my own property, my own car and had many life experiences. If I had keeled over and died at that precise moment, then at least I would have experienced the many things life had afforded me. I'm sure this young man would be unable to say the same.

I struck up a conversation with him and the lady, who, as I had suspected, turned out to be his mother. The young man, whom I shall call Sam, was twenty-five years old and was more experienced in the field of bowel cancer than I was. He had been diagnosed with this dreadful disease some two years earlier, undergone surgery and his subsequent chemotherapy, which had finished over a year before our meeting. He was at the hospital for his first year follow-up scan.

I explained to him, to a degree, that I had just finished treatment and was waiting to undergo my first scan following the completion of my FOLFOX regime. We swapped a few stories and his mother joined in. Our experiences were similar but with subtle differences; for instance, Sam had suffered greatly from 'chemo tan.' His mother explained that following each cycle, Sam's whole body, front and back, from his chin to his toes, turned a pale red in colour. This colouration normally lasted for around twenty-four hours before Sam would turn back to his normal colour. I was shocked and realised that I had possibly experienced this, although minimally. I immediately recalled my foundation moment when my family and I were holidaying in the Lake District a few months previously and my wife had applied the make-up to my top lip, covering the red mark which had appeared from nowhere on that warm, summer evening. I believed this was my 'chemo tan' time. However, it only occurred once and over such a small area. Sam had experienced the same thing, over almost his whole body. It was another example of how people's different experiences of chemotherapy played out.

The time came for my scan. The barium had been swallowed and I presumed my organs were glowing brightly, waiting for their photographs to be taken. Like before, iodine was injected, and like before, the feeling of losing control of my bladder became apparent but this time I knew I hadn't. I left the room, had my cannula removed and dressed myself.

I expected to see Sam still sitting on his chair but he wasn't there, just his mother. My wife and I wished her well and asked her to pass on our best wishes to her son and we left. I only had one more step in this journey to contend with, namely my next appointment with Dr Patel, scheduled for 19th January 2017.

The days leading up to my appointment with the good doctor passed without incident. I was working, although still on a part-time basis and still leaving work when I became tired. After work, I rested and still had to listen to my body.

Winter was in full swing, the days were cold and the dark hours were long. I suffered only from tiredness and had been told this would continue for between six and twelve months. This wasn't a problem. When I was tired, I would rest. It was that simple.

During January, I began to experience pins and needles in my fingertips. It was only in my fingers and not in my toes. I guessed this was the effect of the oxaliplatin and the colder I was, the worse the feelings were. I found I needed to wear gloves more than I had ever done. It seemed the dreaded 'O' had affected the nerves in my fingertips and I believed this would be its lasting result. With what I had experienced during the year of 2016, I realised this was something that I could easily cope with. It seemed a very small price to pay if Mr C had been evicted. My upcoming appointment with the oncologist would confirm whether this would be the case. Deep down, I felt I already knew the results and I felt that together we had defeated 'Him.' 'He' had arrived without invitation and was a very unwelcome and unwanted guest. 'He' had inflicted as much trauma as 'He' could whilst taking up residency. However, 'He' had been removed, firstly by being cut down and secondly by being poisoned. Surely that would be enough – or would it?

The day, 19th January 2017, arrived. My wife and I both met with Dr Patel. We chatted briefly before he told me the news. I believed the news was going to be good but still held within me a sense of caution; after all, you can believe in something completely but still be wrong, can't you?

I had begun this journey almost completely ignorant about bowel cancer. The diagnosis, the treatment, the effects on my body and mind, had all been unknown to me. In turn, my ignorance had bred fear, as the unknown can do. Now, I was not ignorant and had learnt so much on this journey but still that one, underlying fear remained within me. Should Mr C come knocking on my door again I would do my best to keep 'Him' at bay but, I knew that if 'He' wanted to kick that door open, to smash 'His' way back into my life, 'He' had the power to do so. Next time, 'He' may wish to explore further and stay longer. There would be very little I or anyone else would be able to do to stop 'Him'. Having experienced 'Him', it is a fear that will always be with me. The fear that our paths may cross again and our battle recommence – but who would be victorious? We've battled once and my body suffered greatly. I will bear the scars of battle for the rest of my life but I don't want to have to add to those scars.

Dr Patel gave me the news I had wanted and expected.

'There are no signs of cancer in your body,' he said.

With those words, I rose. I grabbed his hand tightly and shook it. I thanked him, with all my heart, for everything he had done for me and my family. He had seen me through the last seven months with great skill, caring and humility, as well as humour when it was needed. He knew that I was grateful beyond words for what he'd done.

My wife and I left the good doctor's office and I was still clutching my little red book close to me. We walked through the waiting room towards the exit. People sat in their chairs waiting for their names to be called and I couldn't help but wonder how many of them were about to begin their own journeys. How many of them were ignorant and fearful of what was ahead of them? It was a question I was unable to answer.

My wife and I walked into the cold evening air outside the hospital. I paused, scouring the darkness, hoping to see the peacock or hear it rustling amongst the bushes. I did not.

We entered the car and were both so happy, so relieved this journey was finally over. My rollercoaster now had its brakes fully applied. I could finally undo my seatbelt and leave this particular rollercoaster behind me, resting upon its final peak.

As we sat in the car I reached over and held my wife tightly to me. I didn't need to tell her how much I loved her, she knew. However, there was a question I did need to ask her. It was a question I had been unable to ask her since my chemotherapy began. It was a question that Mr C had denied me from asking her for so long. Now, 'He' had been forcibly ejected, it was something I could ask. My lips parted and the words flowed from me,

'Fancy a takeaway?'

THE END

EPILOGUE

It has now been almost five years since I underwent surgery. I've had my one- and two-year follow-up CT scans, both of which have thankfully shown no further signs of cancer. I am due my five-year scan very soon which will hopefully bear similar results.

Being diagnosed changed my life. Since recovering, I have given up my career and obtained, shall we say, a less stressful occupation. I decided that life was too short to keep pressurising myself and cancer forced my hand somewhat. It changed the way I viewed life and made me recognise the most important things in life. Mr C focused my thoughts and one Friday I finished work, returned home and spoke to my wife about how I felt. Again, she supported me, my views and the way I was feeling. The weekend passed and Monday morning I gave in my notice and one month later I left my position. I took six weeks off work and had a family holiday in the Caribbean to celebrate my fiftieth birthday.

Since treatment ended, it has not all been a bed of roses. I still suffer with pain in my fingers when they become cold. When the temperature drops, I find myself wearing gloves when most other people aren't. These days I am able to reach deep inside my fridge without difficulty as long as I don't linger there for too long. I still bear the scars physically and mentally of the time my lodger chose to inhabit my body and, undoubtedly, I always will. It was an experience I wouldn't wish on my worst enemy. One which arrived very rapidly and without warning. It really was the case that one day I was healthy and the next I began with the problems which were the start of my journey of some fifteen months.

That journey, for me, is now over. For others, it may not have even begun yet and many are already undertaking their own personal journeys. Inevitably, many of these journeys will end very sadly. 'He' shows little mercy. It doesn't matter who you are, what you have, your gender, sexuality, religious beliefs or what colour skin covers your body. It is impossible to know when or where cancer will strike. What I do know is that the words 'you have cancer' are not, necessarily, a death sentence. Treatments have improved dramatically over the years and continue improving. Remember, if you receive those chilling words, you have a good chance of finishing your journey as you would wish everyone to. Also remember not to ask, 'Why me?' but to ask, 'Why not me?'

ABOUT THE AUTHOR

Anthony Michael's lives on the south coast of England with his wife, son and the family's Basset Hound, Benson. He enjoys cricket and rugby and played both to a high standard as a young man.

He enjoys writing and, although this is his first published work, he is already working on his next book. Further works are planned.

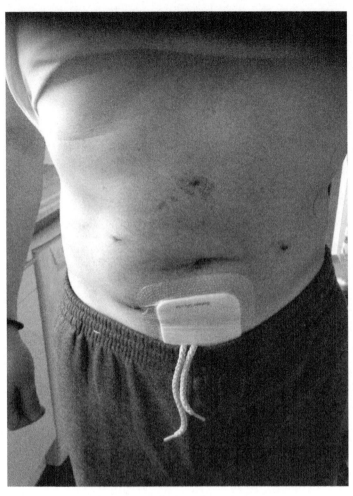

Approximately 1 week post surgery

Your chemotherapy record

This patient is on
CYTOTOXIC CHEMOTHERAPY

INFORMATION FOR PATIENTS

You **MUST** contact the hospital URGENTLY if you feel unwell or develop the following:

- Chest pain or difficulty in breathing
- Temperature greater than 38°C (100°F) or less than 36°C
- Shivering episodes
- Flu-like symptoms
- Gum/nose bleeds or unusual bruising
- Mouth ulcers that stop you eating or drinking
- Vomiting
- Four or more bowel movements a day or diarrhoea

Oncology Unit
Opening hours
Mon to Thurs 9—5
For urgent queries that can't wait until the Unit is open please ring.

N.B. In the event you aren't able to contact our
Unit, please present to your nearest Accident & Emergency Department

Please keep this booklet safe and bring it with you to ALL of your hospital and GP appointments

My Little Red Book

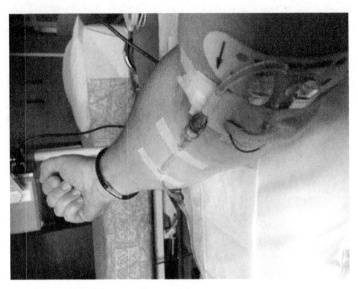

My PICC line and how it was secured

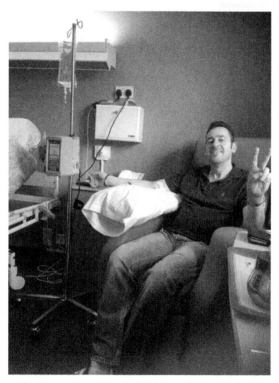

My first chemotherapy cycle 28/6/2016

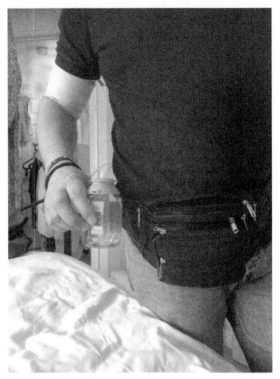

My pump worn for 46 hours after each chemotherapy cycle

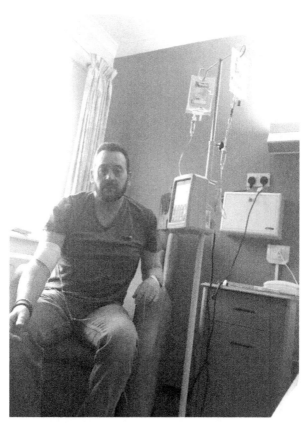

My final chemotherapy cycle 06/12 2016

Printed in Great Britain
by Amazon

66261549R00129